TREADFIT

9 weeks to your ULTIMATE BODY

by Gerard Thorne, BSc, BEd

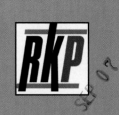

Published by Robert Kennedy Publishing
5775 McLaughlin Road
Mississauga ON
L5R 3P7
Canada

Designed and edited by Wendy Morley
Library and Archives Canada Cataloguing in Publication

Thorne, Gerard, 1963-
        TreadFit : 9 weeks to your ultimate body using a treadmill
or elliptical / Gerard Thorne.

ISBN-13: 978-1-55210-039-4
ISBN-10: 1-55210-039-1

        1. Treadmills (Exercise equipment) 2. Treadmill exercise.
3. Elliptical trainers. I. Title.

GV543.T546 2006   613.7'10284   C2006-906750-3

Distributed in by NBN Books
Head Office
4501 Forbes Blvd.
Suite 200
Lanham, MD 20706

Distribution Center
15200 NBN Way
Blue Ridge Summit, PA 17214

Printed in Canada

TREADFIT

9 weeks to your ULTIMATE BODY

by Gerard Thorne, BSc, BEd

Table of Contents

TreadFit Foreword

by Dr. Clifford Ameduri

When Gerard came to me with his idea to write a book specifically for treadmill users, my first thought was, "What a great idea!" The treadmill is one of the 20th century's greatest inventions. It allows people to get cardiovascular exercise without ever leaving their home. Thus, the treadmill gave an undeniable opportunity to those who would otherwise have a difficult time getting cardio: people who live in northern or rainy climates, or those who feel uncomfortable exercising in front of others.

For years now treadmills have been the most popular piece of home exercise equipment. But they aren't used just in homes. They are used in gyms, health clubs, physiotherapy clinics and rehab centers. Hotels are unlikely to offer a full gym, but they almost always have a treadmill. Be all that as it may, I have never seen a book written for the treadmill user. So my second thought when Gerard came to me with this idea was, "Why didn't I think of that?"

After his work on this book began,

Gerard contacted me once again. "I was thinking of adding elliptical training," he said. Again, a great idea. Elliptical cross trainers are like a combination treadmill, stair climber and cross-country ski machine. They offer great cardiovascular exercise that works the entire body, but – and this is very important – they do not stress the joints! For people who want to get a good workout but have knee or hip troubles, the treadmill can be unforgiving. The elliptical trainer works wonders for them. In fact, the elliptical trainer has been growing so much in popularity that it will likely soon surpass the treadmill.

Whatever the reason you've decided to begin using a treadmill or elliptical trainer – whether you're a true beginner, having never used a piece of exercise machinery before, or you're a fit and healthy young sports enthusiast looking to bring your workouts indoors, or anything in-between, there is no better instructor for you than Gerard Thorne. Gerard has over 25 years' experience in the fitness industry.

He ran the Strength and Conditioning Centre at the YMCA for over 10 years, and has his own personal training company. In addition, he has written over 200 fitness articles for such magazines as *Oxygen* and *Reps!*. In this book, Gerard inspires beginners to get into shape and he inspires those in shape to bring their fitness to new levels. Gerard is well known in the fitness world, not only for his knowledge, but also for his self-deprecating Irish humor. I have no doubt that you'll enjoy the journey this book takes you on, and that you'll come out the other side a fitter, healthier, and happier person.

Of course, we must give the usual caveat. I know you've heard it before, but please take it seriously. Go to your doctor to get the okay before embarking on this, or any other, exercise program. Now go plug in your treadmill or elliptical. It's waiting for you.

In good health,
Clifford Ameduri, MD

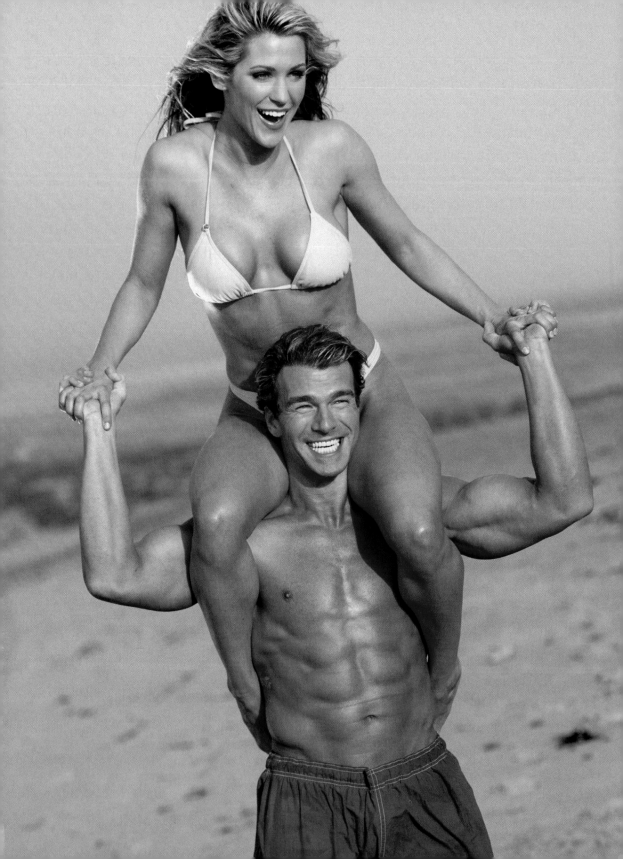

Chapter One

WHY GET IN SHAPE?

You Deserve It!

The number of reasons to get in shape is almost endless. We all have our own reasons for working out. The main thing to remember is that your reasons are just as important as anyone else's. This is not a contest here and you're not being judged. The bottom line is that you decided to do it. Well done and welcome.

For those of you who are still deciding whether or not to take the plunge, take a look at the list at right and see how many of these sound attractive to you. If you find even one, you'll have enough reason to begin an exercise program and begin reaping the many health benefits.

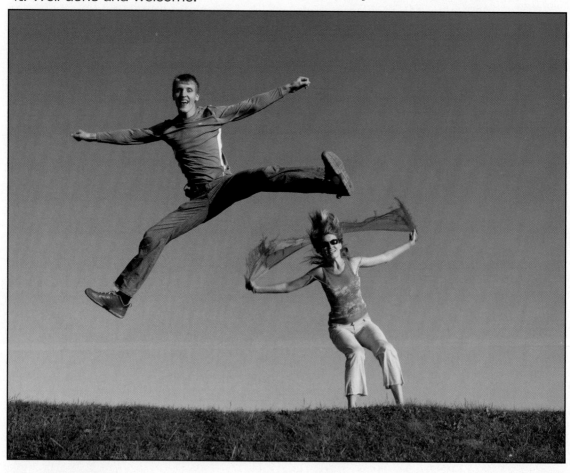

Benefits of Exercise on Cardiovascular Health:

► Helps you lose body fat.

► Improves your body's ability to utilize oxygen and deliver oxygen to your muscle cells.

► Lowers your resting heart rate by enabling your heart to pump more blood per beat. This means your heart doesn't have to work as hard when you are resting.

► Reduces both systolic and diastolic blood pressure. This is vital for people with high blood pressure (called hypertension).

► Lowers your Body Mass Index (BMI) (the ratio of body weight to height). A high BMI rating is linked to cardiovascular disease.

► Lowers LDL (the bad type of cholesterol) and increases HDL (the good type of cholesterol).

► Reduces blood levels of triglycerides (free fatty acids).

► Boosts your immune system.

► Decreases the risk of heart disease.

► Reduces the risk of type II (adult onset) diabetes.

► Decreases the risk of stroke.

Not enough to convince you? Here are some other physical benefits of regular exercise:

Increased muscular strength

Increased physical stamina

Reduced risk of osteoporosis because of increased bone mineral density

Protection against injury

Improved joint function and integrity

Increased muscular endurance

improved balance and coordination

Reduced risk of developing many cancers, including breast cancer

Better sleep

Besides physical benefits, exercise has many psychological benefits:

Reduced anxiety levels

Better stress-coping abilities

Increased self-esteem and confidence

Reduced risk or intensity of depression

Better relaxation

Improved overall quality of life

Improved goal-setting strategies

Increased probability of making better lifestyle choices like quitting smoking

The Cardio-Respiratory System – Your Fitness Highway

The **cardiovascular system** includes the heart and the blood vessels, while the **respiratory system** contains the lungs, larynx and any other parts of the body responsible for absorbing oxygen from the air and expelling the various metabolic waste products, including carbon dioxide.

Blood circulates throughout our bodies in veins and arteries. In simple terms, **arteries carry oxygen-rich blood away from the heart while veins carry oxygen-depleted blood back to the heart.** When the heart pumps it sends oxygen around the body and then brings the deoxygenated blood back to where waste is removed and fresh oxygen picked up. In this respect the heart is really a double pump.

Aerobic vs Anaerobic Respiration

Exercise can be divided into two types of physical activity that perform different functions.

Aerobic exercise involves **sustained activity** that utilizes all the major muscle groups. As your heart and respiratory rates increase, additional oxygen is circulated through the body. This kind of exercise is important for **strengthening your cardiovascular system** and increasing your overall strength and stamina. During aerobic exercise you should bring your heart rate to a level appropriate for your age, then remain at this level for 25 to 30 minutes. For maximum benefit, aerobic exercise should be performed at least three times a week. Examples of aerobic exercise include **walking, jogging, cross-country skiing and swimming.**

Anaerobic means **"without oxygen."** Since the body cannot work for extended periods of time without oxygen, a**naerobic exercise cannot be endured** for long periods of time without a break. The body uses ATP for energy when exercising anaerobically. Some good examples of anaerobic exercise are **sprinting, weight training, and high jumping.**

The type of aerobic exercise you choose depends on your goals, physical condition, and history. While the focus of this book will be on using treadmills and elliptical trainers for aerobic fitness, **it is a good idea to "cross train,"** i.e. alternate different forms of training. This strategy reduces the risk of developing overuse injuries like tendonitis. It also produces a more balanced conditioning effect. Most people will find cross training to be more fun than using only one type of exercise. No matter which types of exercises you choose to perform, you should alternate high-impact exercises (running, tennis, racquetball, squash) with low/moderate impact aerobic exercises (walking, swimming, stair climbing, step classes, rowing, cross-country skiing).

How Long?

The length of your aerobics session depends on such factors as your goals, weekly schedule, and physical condition. For the vast majority of people, 30 to 45 minutes is an acceptable range of time. If your goal is losing body fat and you are in good physical condition, then you can go up to 60 minutes.

What Is Your Target Heart-Rate Zone?

Most experts recommend that, to reap the most rewards from your exercise routine, you pace yourself and monitor your heart rate. For optimal results you should raise your heart rate to what is called the "target heart-rate zone." To calculate your target heart-rate zone, first determine your maximum heart rate, which is 220 minus your age. (This calculation represents a general guideline only.) For example, if you are 35, your maximum heart rate is 220 minus 35, which equals 185. Next, calculate 60 percent and 85 percent of your maximum heart rate. This is the best range for most people during regular exercise. To go back to our example, if you are 35 years old, 60 percent of your maximum heart rate of 185 is 185 x .60 = 111; 85 percent of your maximum heart rate is 185 x .85 = 157. So your target heart-rate zone would be between 111 and 157 beats per minute.

Target Heart Rate Zone.

Age	Target HR Zone	Max HR
20	120-170	200
25	117-166	195
30	114-162	190
35	111-157	185
40	108-153	180
45	105-149	175
50	102-145	170
55	99-140	165
60	96-136	160
65	93-132	155
70	90-128	150
75	87-124	145

Training Zones

Exercise physiologists have divided the target heart-rate zone into five sub-zones:

Healthy Heart Zone (Warm up): *50 to 60 percent of maximum heart rate.*

This is the easiest zone, and probably the best one for people just starting a fitness program. This zone can also be used as a warm up for those in better physical condition. This zone is still effective for decreasing body fat, blood pressure and cholesterol. It also reduces the risk of degenerative diseases and carries a low risk of injury.

Fitness Zone (Fat Burning) *60 to 70 percent of maximum heart rate.*

This zone provides the same benefits as the healthy heart zone, but is slightly more intense and burns more calories.

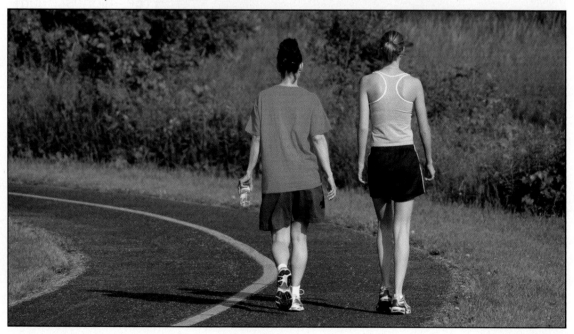

Aerobic Zone (Endurance Training): *70 to 80 percent of maximum heart rate.*
This zone will improve your cardiovascular and respiratory systems and increase the strength and size of your heart. This is your recommended zone if you are training for an endurance event.

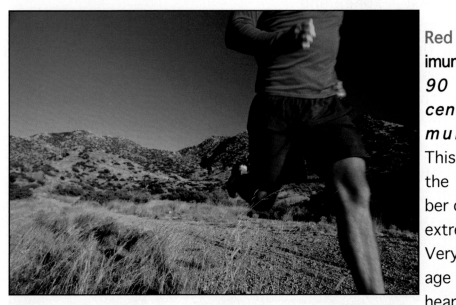

Anaerobic Zone (Performance Training): *80 to 90 percent of maximum heart rate.*
Training in this zone will improve your VO2 max (the highest amount of oxygen you can consume during exercise), and thus will improve your cardio-respiratory system. It also increases your body's ability to tolerate lactic acid, which means your endurance will improve and you'll be able to tolerate fatigue better. Because you are working anaerobically, you cannot continue in this zone for very long.

Red Line (Maximum Effort Zone): *90 to 100 percent of maximum heart rate.*
This zone burns the highest number of calories. It's extremely intense. Very few can manage to bring their heart rate up this high, and those who can do so for only very short periods of time. This zone is potentially dangerous, and is used mainly by competitive athletes. Only train in this zone if you are extremely fit and have been cleared by a physician to do so.

Other Ways to Measure Intensity

While the Target Heart-Rate Zone is probably the most commonly used method to calculate exercise intensity, there are others, including:

1. The "talk test." During your exercise class or cardio session you should be able to talk comfortably. If you can't carry on a normal conversation, you are working too hard.

2. Your perceived exertion level. This simply means how hard the exercise seems to you. The body will usually let you know if you are pushing too hard. If so, listen to it and cool things down a bit.

As time goes on you'll get a better feel for your exercise intensity. We can't emphasize enough that there is no need to kill yourself. Moderate intensity is more efficient and certainly more enjoyable than bringing yourself to the point of collapse. Low-to-moderate intensity is also a good idea when starting back after a layoff, or when you're recovering from an illness or injury. It's also the best level to use if you are significantly overweight.

How often?

Once you're in very good shape, two workouts a week will allow you to maintain your fitness level; but for nearly everyone, three to five sessions a week is optimal. The more often you perform aerobic exercise, the more important it is to cross train, as discussed earlier. Increase your intensity, duration, and frequency gradually. This is especially important if you are sedentary, elderly, overweight, or are recovering from injury or illness. If there is any doubt, go easy, go slowly, and enjoy yourself.

Always warm up and cool down to reduce discomfort and the chance of injury. The easiest way to warm up for aerobic exercise is to perform the exercise at a very low intensity and gradually build up over 5 to 10 minutes.

Likewise, don't suddenly stop the exercise without some sort of cool-down. You run the risk of getting dizzy and/or passing out – especially after being on a treadmill. Many people compare it to getting back on land after being on a ship or boat.

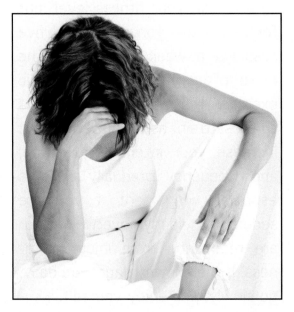

One common misconception is that aerobic exercise tones and firms the muscles. Actually it accomplishes very little toning and firming. In a typical aerobics workout, your active muscles perform hundreds of repetitions with a relatively light resistance placed on them, which is an ineffective toning and firming stimulus. Resistance exercise (weight training) is the only way to shape and tone muscles. This is why we have devoted a separate chapter to the topic later in the book.

Another misconception is that you must exercise at a low intensity to lose fat. Recent research has shown that effective fat loss takes place at any intensity level. There is not enough difference in any of the zones to suggest one over the other. However, increasing intensity does increase total calories burned. That's why the people you see running each day tend to have much lower body-fat levels than those who walk. While healthier and more fit than sedentary people, walkers are likely to still have excess body fat. Hate running? That's okay, you can easily increase the intensity of your walking workout. In fact, at 5 mph running is easier than walking, and at that speed walking burns more calories!

Because aerobic exercise is for the most part repetitive, it does not require a high degree of concentration (although always try to pay attention to technique). Some ways to help pass away the time are listening to music, watching TV, reading a magazine, or chatting to a workout partner (remember, if you can't talk because you are out of breath, you're working too hard).

Your Best Foot Forward with the Right Footwear

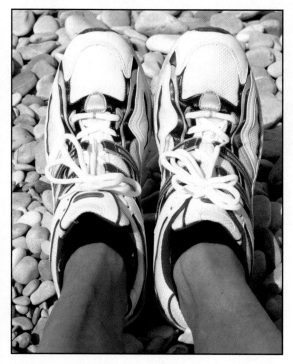

It seems like just yesterday that **people laced up their sneakers whether they were running, walking, shooting baskets, or playing tennis.** The concept of owning more than one pair of athletic shoes and having to decide between cross trainers and runners was nonexistent. Going shopping for a pair of athletic shoes today is like walking into a foreign land. Thanks to such industry trendsetters as Adidas, Reebok and Nike, the multibillion-dollar athletic-shoe industry offers hundreds of styles and brands to choose from. With so many options, you may feel overwhelmed if you haven't done some homework before your shopping trip.

Should you splurge on the latest pair of $250 Nikes or Reeboks? Do you need cross trainers or runners? And where do the Wal-Mart $25 specials fit into all of this? A good rule of thumb is to pay the most attention to comfort, not fancy design. Just because it's denting your wallet more doesn't mean it will give you more protection. And the latest technology won't matter a bit if the shoe hurts your foot in any way.

Take a minute and examine your feet. Generally speaking, your feet fall into one of three categories: low, neutral, or high arched. This is very important to keep in mind when selecting your athletic shoes.

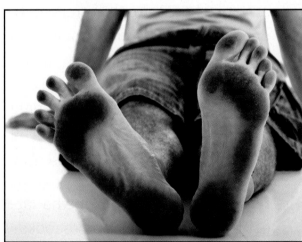

• If you have **neutral-arched feet,** it means your feet are neither overly arched nor overly flat. When you walk or run, your foot hits the ground and rolls slightly to the outside (supination). Then it rolls to the inside as more of your foot makes contact with the ground (pronation). Just before your foot leaves the surface it will roll back toward the outside. For maximum comfort and support, look for shoes with firm midsoles and moderate rear-foot stability.

• If you fall into the **low-arched** category (more commonly called **flat feet**), your foot will have a tendency toward excessive inward rolling (pronation). To make matters worse, this will be exaggerated when running. This condition can lead to knock-knees and some severe knee problems. You want to choose a very stable shoe with good, solid arch support.

• Those with **high arches** will have feet that roll just the opposite way, towards the outside. This can lead to excessive joint and muscle strain as your foot fails to meet the surface properly. Pick shoes with soft midsoles and low rear-foot stability.

One simple technique to determine your foot type is to dip your foot in water and then step on a piece of cardboard. Take a close look at your footprint. Can you see most of your foot? If so you probably have low arches. Conversely, if you see very little of your foot, you most likely suffer from high arches.

You can also look at your old shoes for clues. Place the shoes on a flat surface. Which way do they tilt? If they tilt inward, you most likely have low arches, while tilting outwards indicates high arches. Are the outer edges of your heel and inner edges of the ball of your foot worn down? If so, you probably have neutrally-arched feet. **Don't be afraid to bring your old shoes with you when you go shopping for a new pair.** Any shoe professional worth his salt can determine what you should buy based on the wear of your old shoes. If you have any doubt when buying athletic footwear, be sure to consult a knowledgeable salesperson.

And that brings us back to the $25 Wal-Mart special. While the $250 pair of shoes is not necessarily better than the $125 pair, the $125 pair is definitely better than the $25 pair. Your feet will withstand force seven times your bodyweight when you run. They need at least a modicum of support. Besides it's highly unlikely that you'll find anyone working at your average Wal-Mart, or for that matter any department store, who will be able to tell you which shoes you should buy by looking at your old pair.

Finding the Perfect Fit

In general, the shoe that works for the treadmill will work for the elliptical trainer. Because elliptical trainers are low impact, your shoes will probably last you longer. But don't think it's less important to have a good shoe! You, and your joints, will still be affected if you suffer from overpronation or supination.

Once you're ready to go shopping, look for shoes that fit your feet comfortably, in both length and width. Finding shoes that fit you properly will help you avoid injuries that often result from ill-fitting shoes. Here are a few tips to keep in mind when you shop:

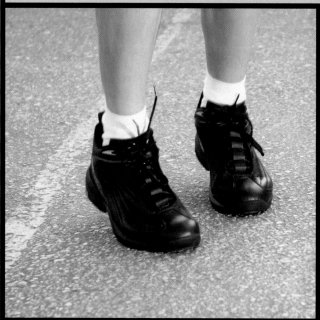

- **Get both feet measured.** Your feet can actually be two different sizes, and you'll want the shoe to fit your largest foot. Your feet expand while bearing your bodyweight, so make sure you're standing when they're measured.
- **Try the shoes on after a workout or at the end of the day.** Your feet tend to swell as the day goes on and will be at their largest during these times.
- **Wear sports socks** similar to those you'll wear during the exercise activity.
- **Try on both shoes** and check the fit. Make sure your heel fits snugly in each shoe and doesn't slip as you walk.
- **Test the shoes for comfort** by walking, or preferably jogging. At a good store the salesperson will watch you jog down the sidewalk or hallway to see if the shoes seem right for you and your step. If the shoes don't feel comfortable right away, take them off and try on another pair. There should be no break-in period for a pair of athletic shoes. They should fit properly from day one.

Rotate your tires

Athletic shoes are like car tires, they wear out. Your shoes may still feel comfortable, but they might not be providing you with the same level of support or shock absorption as when you first bought them. If they tilt excessively inward or outward, it's time to replace them. Likewise, if any part of the sole is worn through, it's time for a new pair. Also, listen to your body. If you start experiencing any new aches and pains, take that as a hint that your shoes may be worn out.

Although this is dependant on how much you weigh and what surface you run on, **shoes should probably be replaced every 300 to 500 miles.** If you run every day or are a competitive walker, you may want to consider having two pairs of identical shoes and alternating them on a daily or weekly basis.

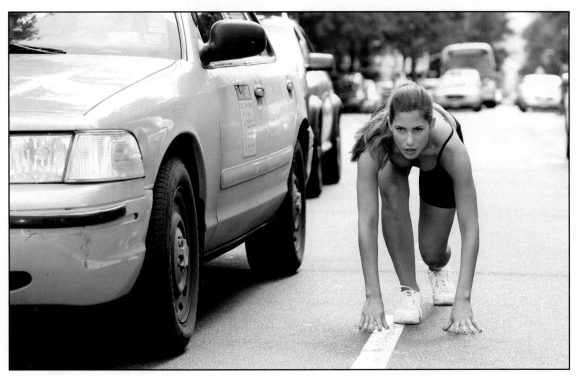

Socks

Like shoes, there are numerous options when it comes to socks. You should probably stay away from cotton, as it absorbs moisture and causes blisters. **Many synthetic socks are made with materials that pull (wick) moisture away from the skin.** You can even get socks with extra thickness in the heel and toe area that gives additional cushioning, helping absorb shock. Another option is wool socks. Wool is highly breathable and keeps your feet comfortable in both cold and warm temperatures.

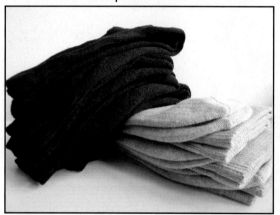

When choosing socks, **make sure they fit your foot.** Socks that are too big will slip, bunch up, and cause blisters. Socks that are too tight can restrict toe movement. Try the socks on with your athletic shoes. The extra padding may make your shoes too tight.

Preventing Blisters

Although blisters don't cause the same drama as injuries, **they can be just as detrimental to your workouts.** One simple little blister can cut your workout short just as quickly as a twisted ankle. But you can prevent blisters.

As just discussed, the proper shoes and socks can go a long ways toward blister prevention. Another little tip is petroleum jelly. **Before a long run, smear a small amount of Vaseline over your entire foot.** This will help reduce friction and prevent blisters from occurring. Another trick is to tape your foot before you head out on your run or hop on the treadmill. This creates a smooth, protective layer between your skin and the area that may flare up and blister. Finally, don't forget an occasional foot massage. They're easy to give to yourself, but they're much better from someone else!

And the Rest

Unless you plan on running in the buff, you'll need a few more items to complete your workout wardrobe. **The simplest and cheapest would be a T-shirt and pair of shorts.** If your workout machine is located in a cold or drafty basement, you might want to upgrade to a sweatshirt and pants. The nice thing about your workout attire is that you have total say in what you wear, whether that's $10 or $1000. Women will want to make sure

they have a good sports bra, no matter what their size. Again, a good sports-clothing store will be able to help you find one appropriate for you. Bouncing breasts may be thrilling for men to watch, but for women they can not only be painful, they can also cause damage to delicate breast tissue.

The great thing about ellipticals and treadmills is that they can be used by anyone to suit any health and fitness goal.

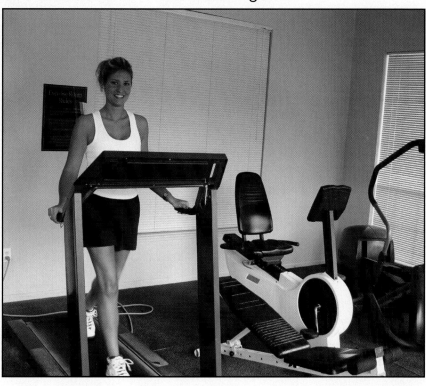

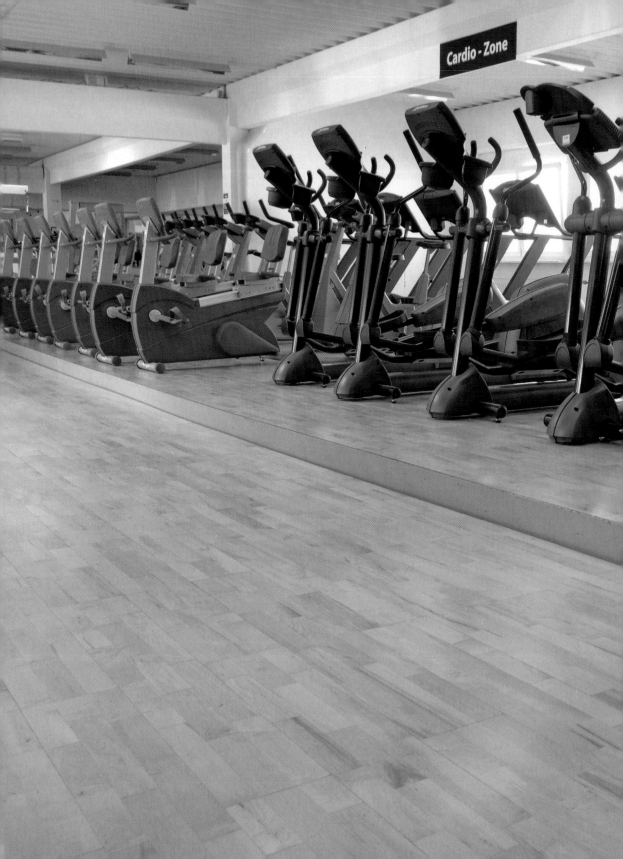

Chapter 2

TREADMILL OR ELLIPTICAL?

No Excuses!

Are you one of those people with a library of excuses for avoiding exercise? Are you too busy with work and family? Is the weather in your area a constant factor, preventing you from exercising outdoors? **Exercising on a treadmill or elliptical trainer is a perfect way to eliminate most excuses** and steer you back on the road to good health and fitness.

Why own a Treadmill?

Research has shown that **the treadmill is the most used piece of indoor fitness equipment,** though the elliptical trainer is fast catching up. Walking is one of the simplest and most effective forms of exercise, and owning your own treadmill makes sticking with a walking or running routine that much easier. If such variables as time, safety, allergies or weather limit your outdoor walking, a treadmill can be a great asset. Do you get the same advantages as with outdoor walking or running? Absolutely! In fact you may even get a better workout since it is much easier to control speed, incline and intensity. The only athletic skill you'll need is the ability to do something you already do on a regular basis – walk. The weather isn't a problem, and to combat boredom just set up your treadmill in front of the television or a large picture window, and put on your walking shoes. You get the benefits of aerobic exercise without leaving the comfort of your own home.

"Winter can't prevent you from getting exercise when you have a treadmill."

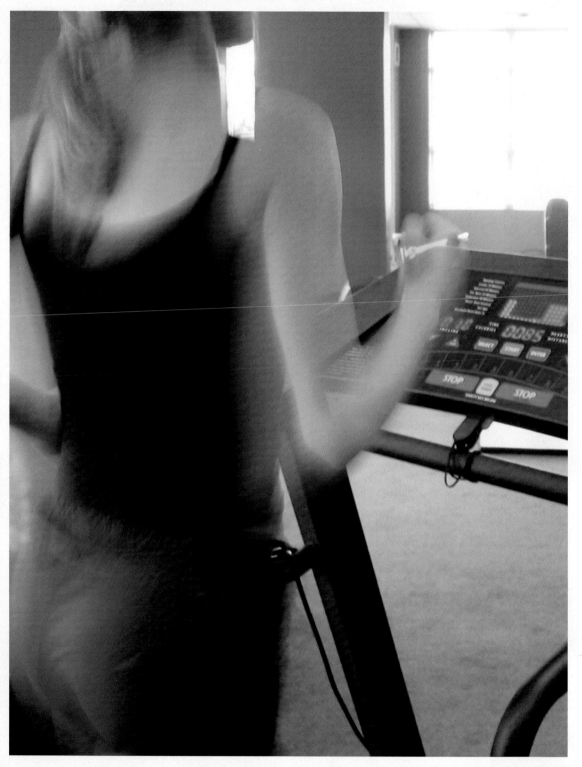

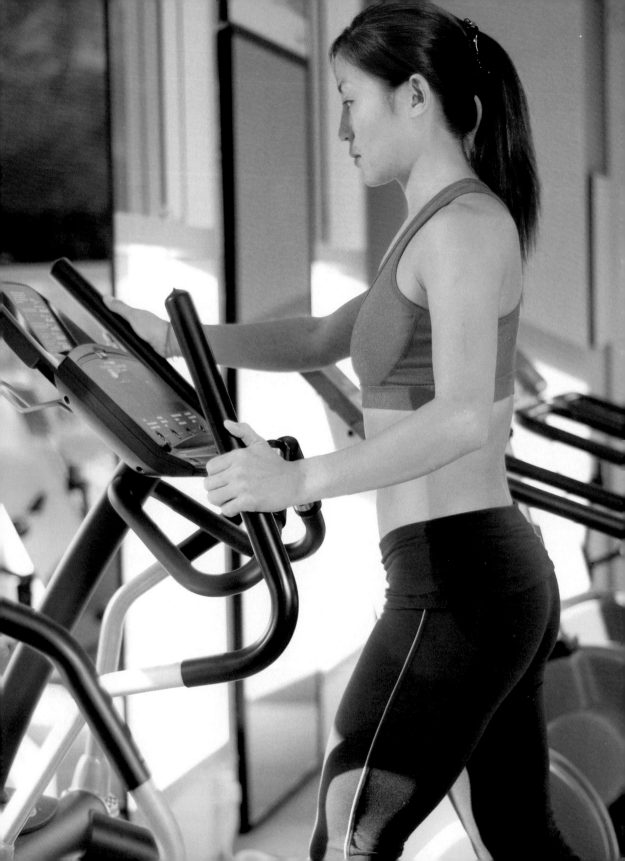

Why own an Elliptical?

Elliptical trainers combine the movements of the stair climber, treadmill and exercise bike into one. **If there were ever a perfect cardio machine, the elliptical trainer would be it.** Not only do they give a great workout, elliptical trainers are easy on the joints, so people who find the pounding of walking or running difficult to bear have no problem in that regard. In addition, ellipticals have moving handles that enable you to also work out your upper body should you choose to. While it can take a workout or two to get used to the motion, there is good reason why ellipticals are catching up to treadmills in popularity.

Choosing your Equipment

Treadmills and ellipticals are easy to set up and make use of, and when used correctly they provide an ideal way to burn calories, control body weight, and enhance your cardiovascular system. But buyer beware! There are countless models to choose from. As this can be a mixed blessing, we're offering you the following tips to make sure you maximize your investment.

Shopping tips

1. Consider your goals and the goals of anyone else in your home before you make your purchase. In most families more than one individual will use the machine. It's important to consider the goals and needs of all possible users. For example, a family might buy a low quality, underpowered treadmill for a 120-pound young woman and her 220-pound father may decide to use it. You may be content to trod along at two or three miles per hour but your athletic teenage son or daughter may regularly run at 10 to 15 miles per hour. If you are just beginning a fitness program, your goals will change along with your improving fitness. Be sure to consider the needs of all possible users, and your future, fit self. Keep in mind that most elliptical trainers are not built for those over 250 pounds.

2. Start your shopping with a trip to an authorized specialty fitness retailer. Make a list of local retailers who specialize in fitness equipment. These dealers are likely to have a knowledgeable staff, higher quality equipment, and – very important but often overlooked – be able to assemble and service your machine effectively. Good dealers will also have relationships with personal trainers to help you start your program.

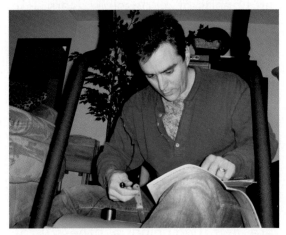

3. Go to the store prepared to truly test the equipment in the manner in which you will be using it. Almost any treadmill will feel adequate if you walk on it for five minutes. It's only when you begin to put a treadmill through its paces by jogging, changing the speed and incline, or using different programs that you will start to notice major differences in quality and comfort.

The range in quality of ellipticals is not so great as with treadmills, but you still want to make sure the machine is adequate for the needs of all. You don't want to find that the pedals don't take your husband's weight. The pedals and arms should feel stable and secure. They should not feel at all loose and you should never feel a list.

4. The heavier the machine's workload, the more durable it must be. You may not need a professional-level piece of equipment, but you don't want it to break down moments after the warranty expires, either. Dress in your actual workout clothes and shoes, and don't hesitate to spend 15 to 30 minutes testing the equipment. A good piece of home cardio equipment is a major investment. Take your time.

Features Your Equipment Should Have:

1. User-friendly console and screen with a large digital readout. Ask yourself, "does the layout make sense?" A salesperson can show you some basics like start and stop, but after the first few minutes the buttons and console should start feeling comfortable.

2. Shock absorption system. Most treadmills have some sort of shock absorption these days, but you must pay attention: When you walk fast

or run, does the treadmill deck feel firm and stable, or loose and unforgiving? It should not feel excessively soft or bouncy, as this type of cushioning can lead to knee injuries down the road. Soft decks also wear out more quickly. On the other side of the coin, you don't want a treadmill that feels like you are running on concrete.

3. Electronic features. Most cardio equipment has a wide spectrum of console features to entice buyers. These range from calories burned to average speed to distance traveled. Electronic features can be both motivating

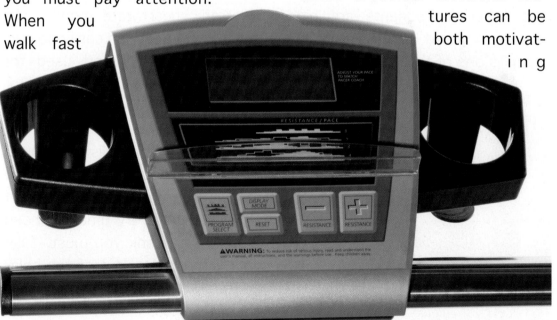

and challenging. Some of the most effective features include interval programs, quick-start modes, and custom-made programs that can be stored for future use. However, **probably the most important feature is a digital clock** that keeps track of how long you have been going, or conversely, how long you still have to go.

4. Motor power. Motor power is one of the most advertised features. But don't be fooled by the "bigger is always better" belief. In reality, a 2.0 horsepower motor is sufficient for virtually any user if the other components are high quality. **A good cooling mechanism** is one of the more important features, because it reduces heat on the motor and the other key components. A large motor with a poor cooling mechanism is a bad combination that will likely result in both poor performance and premature wear and tear.

5. Incline. Inclines vary widely among treadmills, with the usual range being between 0 and 10 to 15 degrees. The larger this range, the more variety you can have in your workouts.

6. Heart-rate monitor. Many treadmills and ellipticals include an electronic heart rate monitor. Of course, this item can easily be purchased separately and used for both your treadmill and outdoor workouts.

7. Drink holder. This may sound trite, but in fact it's important. You do not want to stop and get off your machine every time you need a drink. And drink you must. Take your water bottle out of the holder and have a few sips every couple of minutes.

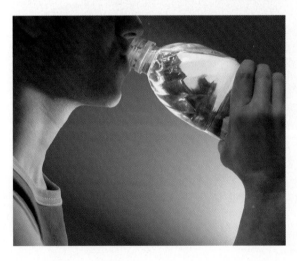

An Investment in your Future

A quality treadmill or elliptical will run you anywhere from $1000 to $10,000 – in general, ellipticals will cost less. Those $250 department-store specials are a waste of money. They will actually cost you more money in the long run in parts and labor – even hospital bills. Make sure you purchase a solid, strong machine that will last you and your family for years to come.

Remember. Paying for Quality Now will Pay of in Health for Years to Come.

Take your time and choose wisely. One of the surest ways to buy quality is to go with a manufacturer that has a history of quality. Go with a company that makes equipment for health clubs and other high-use facilities like corporate gyms and university settings. A company whose equipment is used dozens of times a day in a commercial setting is likely to make a household unit that will stand up well.

Better Treadmill Companies:
- Smooth
- Precor
- Trimline
- Proform
- Life Fitness
- Landice

Better Elliptical Companies:
- Smooth
- Precor
- Schwinn

(according to www.consumersearch.com, a Web site that "reviews the reviews.")

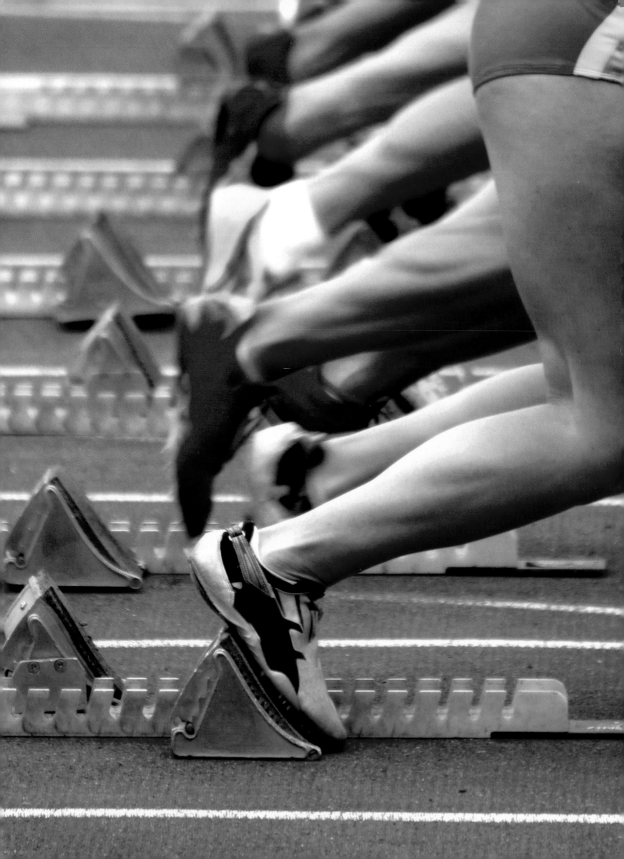

Chapter 5

9 Weeks
to your
Ultimate Body

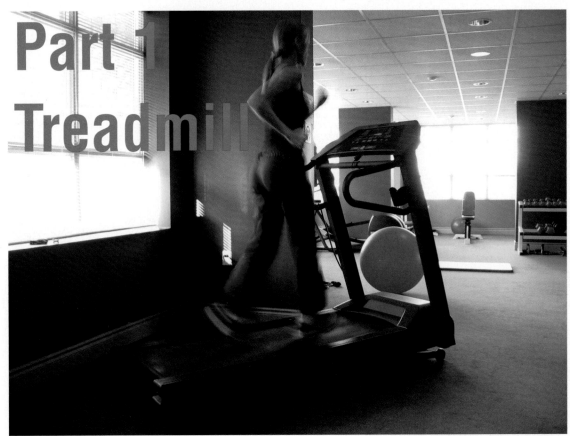

Part 1
Treadmill

The Basics

Warm-up (5 minutes)

Walk slowly with a normal gait for about one minute at about 2 mph. Walk on your toes for 30 seconds, then switch to your heels for 30 seconds. Repeat the toe and heel walking for another 30 seconds each. Raise the incline to 5 or 6 degrees, and stretch your legs by taking longer strides for about one minute. Lower the incline to 0, and speed up to 2.5 to 3 mph for another minute.

Cool down (5 minutes)

At the end of your walk, reduce your speed to 2.5 to 3.5 mph, and walk for 2 to 3 minutes. Then reslow down to 1.5 to 2.5 mph, and walk for an additional 2 more minutes.

Stretch

To avoid having your calves tighten, try this stretch: Stand on the edge of a step and gently lower one heel. Hold for 45 to 60 seconds. Switch to the other leg and repeat.

Strength Moves

The following exercises will help improve your strength for your treadmill workouts. Walk at a very slow speed (about 0.5 to 1 mph) for the first two exercises, then stop the treadmill for the third. If you have time, repeat the whole three-minute sequence. As you get fitter, you can increase the speed, but stay at or below 2 mph.

Side Stepping

With the treadmill moving slowly and your right hand on the console, turn to the left so your right shoulder is facing forward. As the belt moves your feet to the left, step your right foot to the right, and then step your left foot to the right. Continue side-stepping for 30 seconds. Then turn around and do this exercise facing the opposite direction for 30 seconds. This movement is great for the inner and outer thighs and hips.

Lunge Stepping

Holding the front rail, let the belt take your feet back until your arms are extended, then take a large step forward with your right leg. Bending your right knee, lower your left knee toward the belt, then press off with your left foot and stand back up. Continue by stepping forward, alternating legs, for 30 seconds.

Squats

Stop the treadmill and straddle the belt so you're standing on the frame. With your hands lightly resting on the front rail, sit back as if in a chair, but don't extend your knees past your toes. Press into your heels, and stand back up. Repeat 12 times.

Here is a program that will bring you from walking to running – and in your best shape ever – in nine weeks. This program has you doing your cardio four times each week. Keep in mind that the best results will come if you have a good diet and do a weight-training workout at least twice per week.

Please make sure you warm up and cool down before and after every single workout.

The cooldown should take a little longer as your workouts become more intense. So during week one your cooldown will last five minutes, slowing down twice. By the end of the ninth week you will slow down to a jog for a couple of minutes, then do the walking cool down. This will add an extra two minutes to your workout.

Week 1

Increase walking speed

Day 1: Warm up • walk for 20 minutes at 3 mph • cool down

Day 2: Warm up • walk for 20 minutes at 3.3 mph • cool down

Day 3: Warm up • walk for 20 minutes at 3.6 mph • cool down

Day 4: Warm up • walk for 20 minutes at 4.0 mph • cool down

Week 2
Start to jog

Day 1: Warm up • walk 4.0 mph for 2 minutes, jog 5 mph for 30 seconds ... continue this walk/jog sequence for 20 minutes • cool down.

Day 2: Warm up • walk 2.5 minutes, jog 45 seconds ... continue this sequence for 20 minutes • cool down.

Day 3: Warm up • walk 3 minutes, jog 1 minute ... continue this sequence for 20 minutes. Cool down.

Week 3
Work on an incline

Day 1: Warm up • set incline to 2 percent • walk/jog as in week 2 day 4 • cool down.

Day 2: Warm up • set incline to 3 percent • walk/jog as before • cool down.

Day 3: Warm up • set incline to 4 percent • walk/jog as before • cool down.

Day 4: Warm up • set incline to 5 percent • walk/jog as before • cool down.

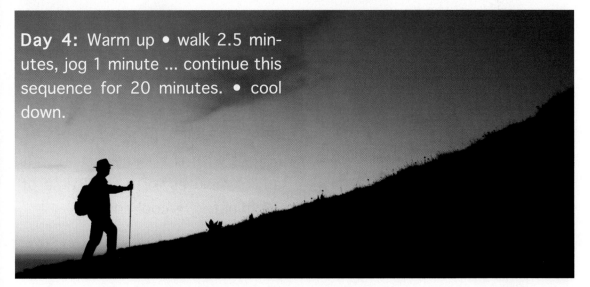

Day 4: Warm up • walk 2.5 minutes, jog 1 minute ... continue this sequence for 20 minutes. • cool down.

Week 4

Increase your time

Day 1: Warm up • walk/jog as before with the same incline, but add 2 minutes for a total time of 22 minutes • cool down.

Day 2: Warm up • walk/jog as before but add 2 minutes for a total time of 24 minutes • cool down.

Day 3: Warm up • walk/jog as before but add 3 minutes for a total time of 27 minutes • cool down.

Day 4: Warm up • walk/jog as before but add 3 minutes for a total time of 30 minutes. • cool down.

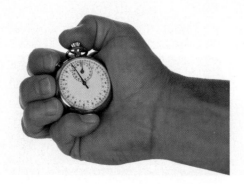

Week 5

Improve overall fitness

Day 1: Warm up • keep the incline at 5 percent, the walking speed at 4.0 mph and the jogging speed at 5 mph, but walk 2 minutes and jog 2 minutes for a total of 30 minutes • cool down.

Day 2: Warm up • keep walking/jogging as before, but increase the incline to 6 percent . Your incline will remain at 6 until the end of this program.• cool down.

Day 3: Warm up • keep walking/jogging as before, with the incline at 6 percent, but add 2 minutes for a total of 32 minutes • cool down.

Day 4: Warm up • walk/jog as before with the same incline, but add 3 minutes for a total time of 35 minutes. • cool down.

Week 6
Increase jogging time

Day 1: Warm up • keep incline at 6 percent, but walk for 1.5 minutes and jog for 2 minutes for a total of 35 minutes • cool down.

Day 2: Warm up • keep incline and sequence the same, but add two minutes for a total of 37 minutes. • cool down.

Day 3: Warm up • keep incline and length of workout the same, but walk for 1 minute and jog for 2. • cool down.

Day 4: Warm up • keep incline and sequence the same, but add 3 minutes for a total of 40 minutes • cool down.

Week 7
Get ready to run

Day 1: Warm up • try to jog all the way through 40 minutes at an incline of 6. Walk at times if you must. • cool down.

Day 2: Warm up • jog for 40 minutes at a 6 percent incline • cool down.

Day 3: Warm up • jog 5 mnutes at 5 mph, run 30 seconds at 7 mph. Continue this sequence for 40 minutes. • cool down.

Day 4: Warm up • jog 5 minutes and run for 45 seconds ... continue sequence for 40 minutes • cool down.

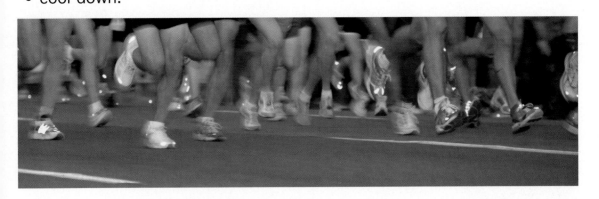

Week 8
Getting there...

Day 1: Warm up • jog 5 minutes and run for 1 minute ... continue sequence for 40 minutes • cool down.

Day 2: Warm up • jog for 5 minutes and run for 1.5 minutes ... continue sequence for 40 minutes. • cool down.

Day 3: Warm up • jog for 4 minutes and run for 2 minutes ... continue sequence for 40 minutes • cool down.

Day 4: Warm up • jog for 4 minutes and run for 2 minutes • cool down.

Week 9
Now you're a runner!

Day 1: Warm up • jog for 3 minutes, run for 3 ... continue sequence for 40 minutes.• cool down.

Day 2: Warm up • jog for 2 minutes, run for 3 ... continue sequence for 40 minutes • cool down.

Day 3: Warm up • jog for 1 minute, run for 4 ... continue sequence for 40 minutes. • cool down.

Day 4: Warm up • run for 40 minutes. • cool down.

References
1) Marianne McGinnis, 12-Week Treadmill Workout, Indoor fat-blasting walking routines for every body.
http://www.prevention.com/cda/feature2002/0,2479,s1-6545,00.html

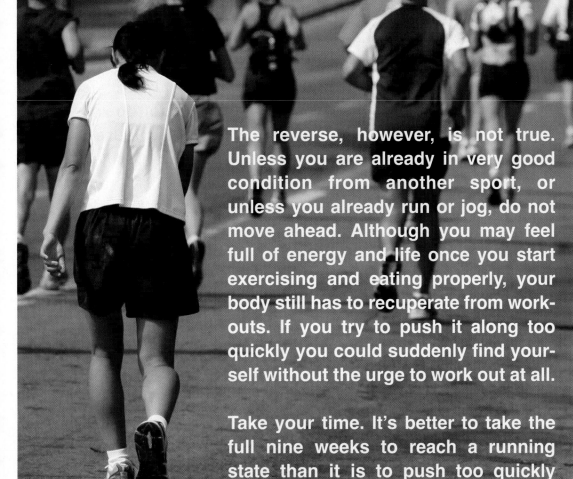

There you have it, a program that will take you from walking to running in nine weeks. Please keep in mind that you must listen to your own body. If you do not feel ready to take the next progressive step, stay where you are for an extra day or two. When you are ready, move to the next progression.

The reverse, however, is not true. Unless you are already in very good condition from another sport, or unless you already run or jog, do not move ahead. Although you may feel full of energy and life once you start exercising and eating properly, your body still has to recuperate from workouts. If you try to push it along too quickly you could suddenly find yourself without the urge to work out at all.

Take your time. It's better to take the full nine weeks to reach a running state than it is to push too quickly through the first three weeks only to quit because you've overtrained.

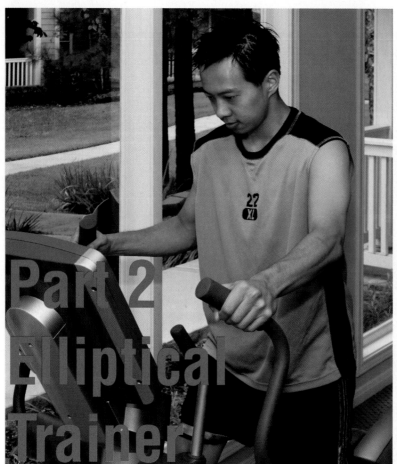

Part 2 Elliptical Trainer

The Basics

Every time you work out you must be sure that you warm up, cool down, and stretch afterwards. This will help you avoid injury and will make your workout more effective.

Warm-up (5 minutes)

Hop onto your elliptical, make sure your feet are placed properly, and start moving. Pump the handles to get your upper body warmed up. You can warm up without any resistance at all when you are beginning. Once you become accustomed to the machine and to getting exercise, warm up on a level 2 or 3. Some programs have a warm-up built in.

Cool down (5 minutes)

Again, some programs will have a cooldown built in. Make sure yours lasts for five minutes, or you can extend it manually. Otherwise, bring the machine down to a level 2 or 3 and stay there for five minutes once you've finished your workout.

Stretch

It's by far best to stretch after you have cooled down. Your muscles, tendons and ligaments are all nice and warm and pliable. Stretch your calves, quads, hamstrings, hip flexors, pecs, back, shoulders, and arms.

This program is set up for someone working out four times per week. It assumes that the trainer is a beginner with no health troubles.

Please keep in mind that this is only a guideline. Do not push yourself past your own capabilities! If you are not ready to move on, stay where you are for another couple of workouts.

If you try a workout and feel it is stressing you too much, go back to the previous one. You will never get into great shape if you begin to dread your workouts or you get an injury.

Levels of difficulty vary from machine to machine. Level 5 may seem easy on one machine and difficult on another. Use your heart rate and the way you feel as your guide. Okay, here is a program that will take you from beginner to old hat in nine weeks.

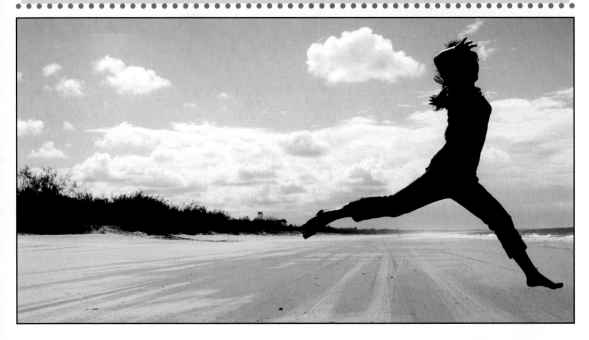

Week 1
Getting the hang of It

Day 1: Get comfortable on your machine. It can take a little work to get the movement down right, so that will be the concentration for the first day. Before turning on the machine, start moving the

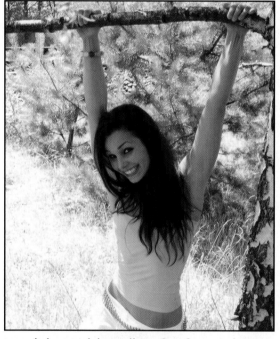

pedals and handles Go for at least a couple of minutes until you feel quite comfortable with the movement. Now turn on the machine. Set your elliptical trainer on the "Manual" program. Set it to a low level – say, level 2 or 3. Continue on at this pace for 20 minutes. Concentrate on keeping your movements between your legs and your arms comfortable and in sync.

Day 2: You should be feeling a little more at ease today. Warm up for five minutes, anywhere from level 0 to level 2. Then go up to level 4. Stay there for 20 minutes, then cool down at level 2 for five minutes. If you find it too much to keep your arms going the whole time, use them intermittently.

Day 3: Warm up for five minutes. Go up to level 4 for 20 minutes. Cool down for five minutes.

Day 4: Warm up for five minutes. Go up to level 4 for four minutes, then reverse your gait. Don't worry about speed, just go backwards for one minute. Repeat sequence of four minutes forward and one minute backward until the 20 minutes is up. Cool down for five minutes.

Week 2
Increase resistance

Day 1: Warm up for five minutes. Go to level 4 for two minutes, to level 5 for one minute, then switch and go backwards for one minute. Continue sequence for 20 minutes. Cool down for five minutes.

Day 2. Warm up for five minutes. Go to level 4 for one minute, level 5 for one minute, level 4 for another minute, level 5 for one minute, then backwards for one minute. Continue this sequence for 20 minutes. Cool down for five minutes.

Day 3: Warm up for five minutes. Go to level 5 for four minutes, then backwards for one minute. Continue this sequence for 20 minutes. Cool down for five minutes.

Day 4: Warm up for five minutes. Go to level 5 for three minutes,

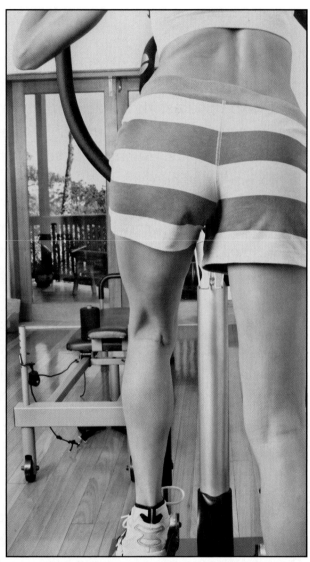

level 6 for one minute, then backwards for one minute. Continue this sequence for 20 minutes. Cool down for five minutes.

Week 3
Increase time and resistance

Day 1: Warm up for five minutes. Go to level 5 for two minutes, level 6 for two minutes, then backward for one minute. Continue this sequence for 22 minutes. Cool down for five minutes.

Day 2: Warm up for five minutes. Go to level 5 for two minutes, level 6 for two minutes, then backward for one minute. Continue this sequence for 25 minutes. Cool down for five minutes.

Day 3: Warm up for five minutes. Go to level 5 for one minute, level 6 for two minutes, then backward for one minute. Continue this sequence for 27 minutes. Cool down for five minutes.

Day 4. Warm up for five minutes. Go to level 5 for one minute, level 6 for two minutes, then backward for one minute. Continue this sequence for 30 minutes. Cool down for five minutes.

Week 4
Add some excitement

Day 1: Warm up for five minutes. Go to the "Interval" program on level 6. Follow this program for 30 minutes. Cool down for five minutes.

Day 2: Warm up for five minutes. Go to the "Interval" program on level 6. Follow this program for 30 minutes. Cool down for five minutes.

Day 3: Warm up for five minutes. Go to the "Hill" program (sometimes called "Himilayan" or "Mountain" on level 6. Follow this program for 30 minutes. Cool down for five minutes.

Day 4: Warm up for five minutes. Go to the "Hill" program on level 6. Follow this program for 30 minutes. Cool down for five minutes.

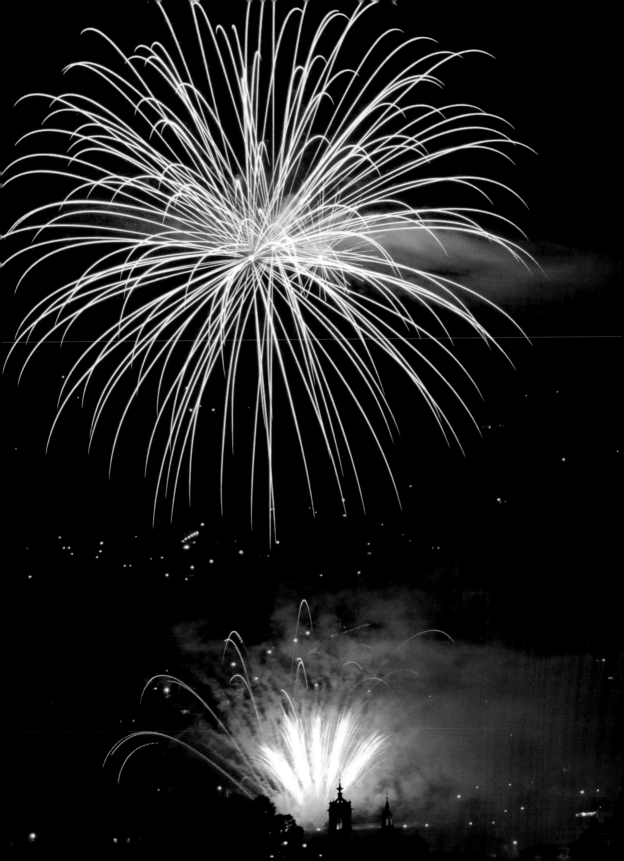

Week 5
"Fartlek" training

Day 1: Warm up for five minutes. Set machine on the "Manual" program. Go to level 6 for one minute, then down to level 2 for 30 seconds. Go to level 7 for 30 seconds, then down to level 2 for 30 seconds. Go to level 8 for 30 seconds, then level 2 for 30 seconds. Keep up like this for a total of 30 minutes, paying close attention to the way you feel. If you need to stay at the lower level for longer, go ahead. If you can't quite make level 8, that's fine ... don't do it. But you want to go up to a challenging level for 30 seconds and then an easy level for 30 seconds. Cool down for five minutes.

Day 2: Warm up for five minutes. Do the fartlek training just as you did on day 1, but attempt to bring the hard-training segments to 40 seconds a time. You can keep the "rest" segments at 30 seconds or increase them to 40 seconds if you feel that it's necessary. Do this for 30 minutes. Cool down for five minutes.

Day 3: Warm up for five minutes. Do fartlek training for 30 minutes – hard training for 50 seconds, rest segments for as long as necessary. Cool down for five minutes.

Day 4: Warm up for five minutes. Do fartlek training for 30 minutes – attempt to bring your hard-training segments up to one minute. Again, your rest segment should be as long as is necessary to get your strength back.

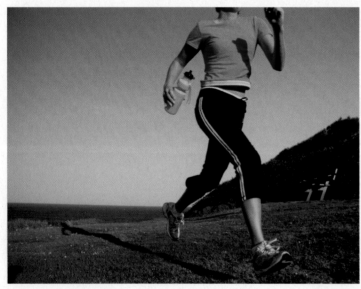

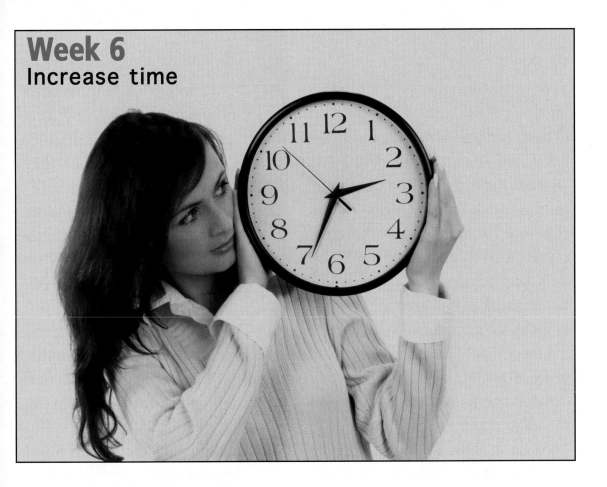

Week 6
Increase time

Day 1: Warm up for five minutes. Set machine on the "Interval" program on level 6. Go for 32 minutes. Cool down for five minutes.

Day 2: Warm up for five minutes. Set machine on the "Interval" program on level 6 for 35 minutes. Cool down for five minutes.

Day 3: Warm up for five minutes. Set machine on the "Interval" program on level 6. Go for 37 minutes. Cool down for five minutes.

Day 4: Warm up for five minutes. Set machine on the "Interval" program on level 6. Go for 40 minutes. Cool down for five minutes.

Week 7

Trying new programs

(These programs may have different names on your machine.) The "Pyramid" program is the one that gets steadily more difficult until the peak, at which point the difficulty steadily decreases until the end. The "Random" program is just like it sounds; the level of difficulty goes up and down in a random manner. The "Cascade" program goes steadily up, then steadily down, then steadily up, then steadily down. "Heart Rate Hill" goes up in difficulty quite steadily until cooldown, when it drops off suddenly. Please keep in mind that a level you may find simple on some programs will be difficult on others. Adjust accordingly.

Day 1: Warm up for five minutes. Set machine on the "Pyramid" program on level 6. Go for 40 minutes. Cool down for five minutes.

Day 2. Warm up for five minutes. Set machine on the "Random" program on level 6. Go for 40 minutes. Cool down for five minutes.

Day 3: Warm up for five minutes. Set machine on the "Cascade" program on level 7. Go for 40 minutes. Cool down for five minutes.

Day 4: Warm up for five minutes. Set machine on the "Heart Rate Hill" program. Cool down for five minutes.

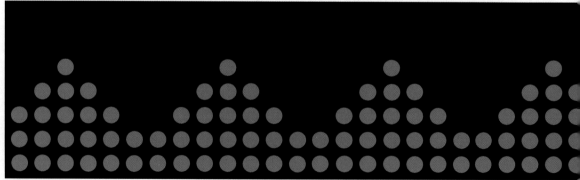

Week 8
Your faves

Day 1: Warm up for five minutes. Set your elliptical on whichever program you prefer, on a level that is challenging but not excessive. (Don't pick one just 'cause it's easy!) Go for 40 minutes. Cool down for five minutes.

Day 2: Warm up for five minutes. Set your elliptical on the same program you used for Day 1, but set it one level higher. Try to complete the whole 40 minutes on this level, but bring it down if you find it too hard. Cool down for five minutes.

Day 3: Warm up for five minutes. Set your elliptical on another of your preferred programs. Set it on a level that is slightly challenging but not excessive. Go for 40 minutes. Cool down for five minutes.

Day 4: Warm up for five minutes. Set your elliptical on the same program as Day 3, but one level higher. Again, try to stay on this level for the whole 40 minutes, but if that is too difficult, bring the level down. Cool down for five minutes.

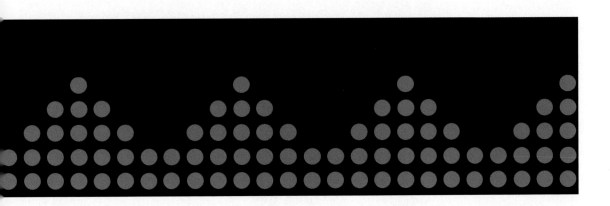

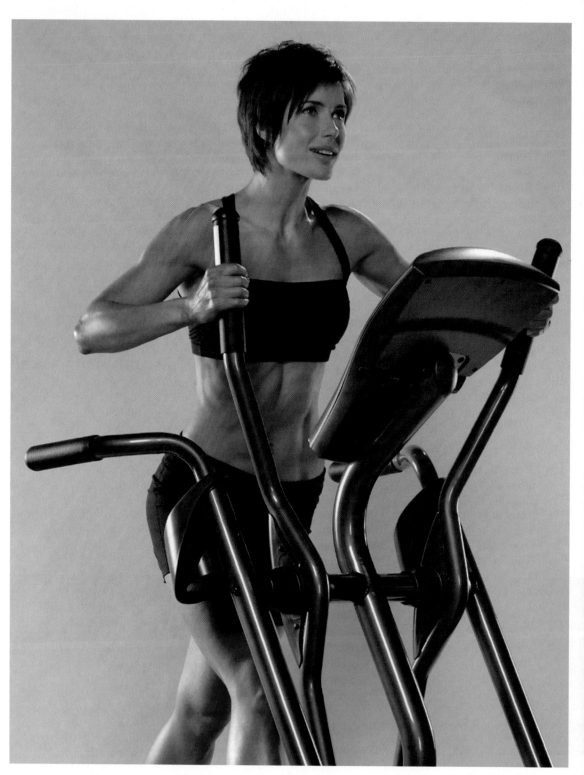

Week 9
Fartlek training

Day 1: Warm up for five minutes. Set machine on "Manual" at level 6 for one minute, then bring it down to level 3 for one minute. Bring the level up to 7 for one minute, then down to 4 for one minute. Bring the level up to 8 for one minute, then 2 for one minute. Keep this up for 40 minutes, playing close attention to how you feel. Cool down for five minutes.

Day 2: Warm up for five minutes. Set machine on "Manual" at level 6 for one minute, then bring it down to level 3 for one minute. Bring it up to 7 for one minute, then down to 4 for one minute. Bring it up to level 8 for one minute, then level 4 for one minute. Keep this up for 40 minutes, paying close attention to how you feel. Try to push one or two difficult levels for 10 seconds more. Cool down for five minutes.

Day 3: Warm up for five minutes. Set machine on "Manual" at level 7 for one minute, then bring it down to level 3 for one minute. Continue as on previous days, bringing your levels up to challenge you then down for a rest, but 1) try to push two difficult levels for 10 seconds more, and 2) try to go up to level 9 for one minute. Keep this up for 40 minutes. Cool down for five minutes.

Day 4: Warm up for five minutes. Set machine on "Manual" at level 7 for one minute, bring it down to level 4 for one minute. Continue as on previous days, but try to keep your levels slightly higher. Try level 10. However, please make sure you do not go overboard. If you have had a very difficult level, make sure to set a very low level to recover before going back up again. Do this for 40 minutes. Cool down for five minutes.

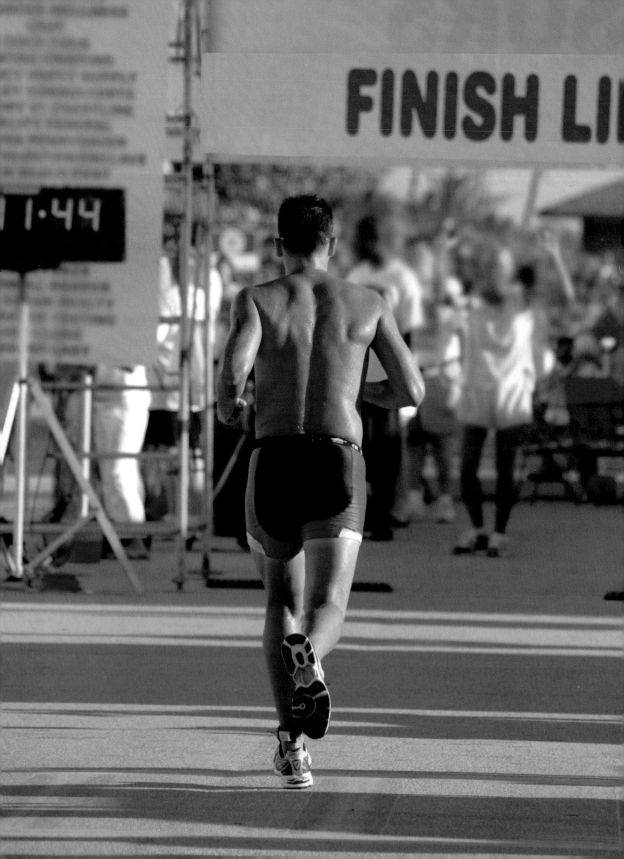

Chapter Three

START MOVING!

Mastering Good Technique

You'll only keep working out if you enjoy what you're doing. How many times have you seen runners plodding along as if they were in pain? Chances are, those runners are not using proper technique. Proper technique will help make your workouts more enjoyable, and that will keep you coming back.

Proper technique is vital for:

1. Efficiency.

When you move efficiently, you eliminate unnecessary movement and hence wasted motion. As you run, try to produce a straight-ahead movement rather than side-to-side motion.

2. Reducing the chance of injury.

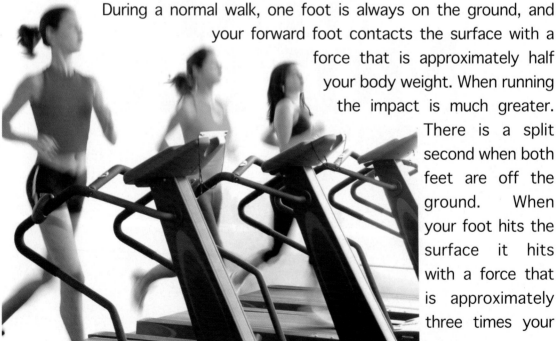

During a normal walk, one foot is always on the ground, and your forward foot contacts the surface with a force that is approximately half your body weight. When running the impact is much greater. There is a split second when both feet are off the ground. When your foot hits the surface it hits with a force that is approximately three times your bodyweight. If your technique is not correct, that force can end up causing you injury.

Tall and Relaxed

The most important concept when running or working out on an elliptical is to remain tall and relaxed. **Keeping your posture erect produces less stress on the joints.**

Drill Techniques To Improve Running

To maximize your running technique you can break the different parts of the run down into a series of drills. A running drill mimics technically sound running form, such as upright posture, proper sway of the arms, and correct knee movement and leg action. Another benefit of running drills is that they help to strengthen the specific muscle groups needed for efficient running, especially the muscles of the thighs, hamstrings, hips, and calves.

The running technique drill outlined next involves marching (walking). Once mastered, it can be incorporated into your running motion.

You're in the Army Now!

The marching drill provides an excellent starting point for beginners who wish to practice the finer points of their running technique. Start out slowly but speed it up as your balance and stability improve. The great thing about this drill is that it allows you to focus on maintaining good posture, synchronizing your arms and legs and stabilizing your movement.

Here are a few tips:
1. **Start out slowly** by walking on the balls of your feet.
2. **Try to prevent your heels from touching the ground** during this exercise.
3. **Use short steps,** approximately 12 to 18 inches in length.

To begin, raise your right knee to

hip level (so that your thigh is parallel to the ground) on each step. Try to keep your ankle directly under or slightly behind the elevated knee. As your body passes over the left foot during the stride, rise on the toes of the left foot and extend the left knee. Try to keep your chin and torso upright and move your arms slowly and in rhythm with the stride.

Keep in mind that this is a practice drill, so **focus on correct posture, arm movement and whole-body balance.** Perform the drill in a slow and controlled manner. The marching drill emphasizes a proper knee lift, upright posture, and a coordinated arm swing, all of which are essential components of proper running.

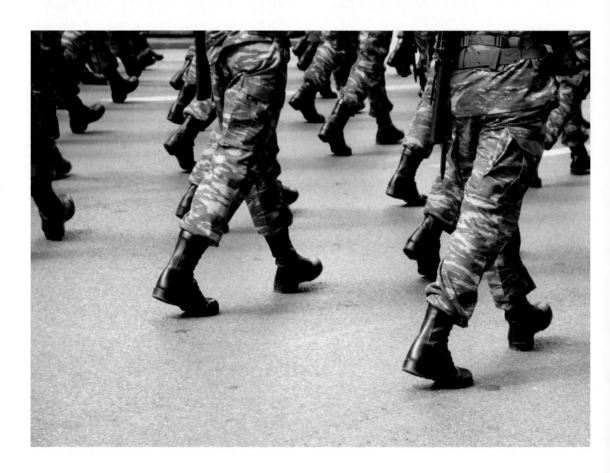

The Do's

• Do change quickly from one leg to the other.

• Do try to raise your ankle straight up under the hips.

• Do keep your support time short.

• Do keep your body-weight on the balls of your feet.

• The ankles should be fixed at the same angle

• Do keep shoulders, hips and ankles along one vertical line.

• Do keep the stride length and range of motion constant.

The Don't's

• Don't touch the ground with your heels; keep heels slightly above the ground.

• Don't shift your weight to the toes or try to pull your ankle up; your weight is on ball of the foot.

• Try not to move the ankles back and forth.

• Don't let your knees and thighs move too far apart, forward, or backward during the stride.

• Concentrate more on lifting than landing.

• Don't land on the toes.

• Don't push off with the toes.

Taking the Plunge ...

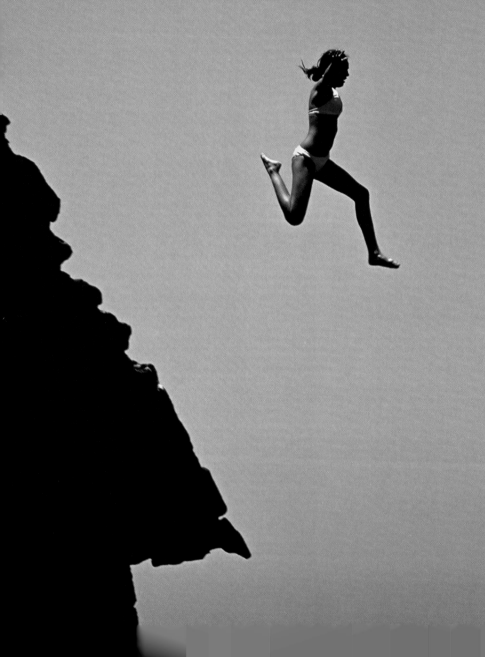

And Now We Begin

Okay, it's now **time to boldly step onto the machine.** We recommend that you start out at a fairly easy pace for 15 to 20 minutes. How fast you go should be determined by your heart rate. Right now you want to stay at the bottom of your training range, between 60 and 70 percent of your maximum predicted heart rate. This will allow you to work out without tiring too quickly. Your training range is 60 to 85 percent of your theoretical maximum heart rate based upon your age.

The formula for calculating your training range is:
220 minus your age = maximum predicted heart rate.

Between 60 and 85 percent of that figure is the range a healthy person wants to be working in to receive cardiovascular benefits.

To determine your heart rate you need to take your pulse. You can **take your pulse by placing the index and middle fingers of one hand on your opposite wrist, just below the base of your thumb.**

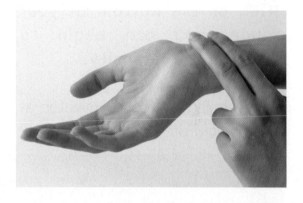

Count the beats for 10 seconds and multiply by six, or count for 15 seconds and multiply by four. **If math is not your strong suit, you can wear a wireless heart rate monitor.** The transmitter is worn around the chest next to the skin. You wear the receiver on your wrist like a watch. There are basic models available for less than $100 from mail-order catalogs that sell biking or running gear. Sporting goods stores will carry them too.

Once you are accustomed to exercising for 20 minutes, work up to 30 minutes, and then 40 to 45 minutes. **Once you become comfortable working out for 45 minutes at 60 percent MHR, or the bottom of your range, you can begin to increase the intensity.**

Try warming up for 10 minutes at the bottom of your training range,

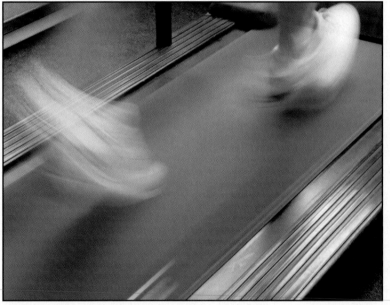

and then **increase the speed until you reach 75 percent MHR. Stay there for a couple of minutes, and then drop the** **speed back down until you again are at 60 percent.** This is known as interval training, and is a great way to build up your cardio capacity over a short period of time. Try a little interval training two or three times during your walk. Over a couple of weeks, slowly increase the length of time you do your cardio workout and the pace at which you do it.

On a treadmill, you can walk up an incline to increase the intensity of your workout without having to walk faster. On the elliptical trainer you will want to use the resistance to increase your intensity. Every couple of weeks, increase the resistance level by one. If, during your workout, you find it too difficult, you can decrease by one, but each workout try to stay at the increased level for longer.

Keep Things Interesting

One of the great things about an elliptical trainer is that it usually

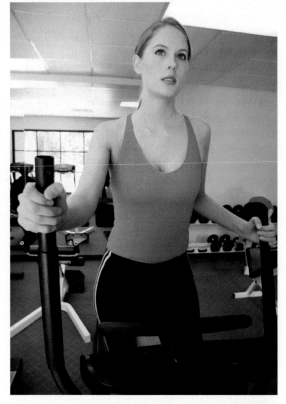

has lots of great programs to keep things interesting. Please, make sure you try these different programs. In addition, make sure you vary your speed. Do a little "fartlek" training. Fartlek means "speed play" in Swedish. In fartlek training you vary your speed, going all out, and then calming down. This is similar to interval training, though a little less regimented. Ellipticals also go backwards. This can take a little while to get used to, but once you do you will find a) your fitness improves, as you are using different muscles and b) it helps your enthusiasm. You could go forward for two minutes, backward for one.

While some treadmills also have programs, a great many of them do not. One disadvantage with treadmills is that it's fairly easy to lose touch with your creative side as soon as you step onto that revolving black conveyor belt. Day after day it's 30 minutes at three miles per hour at five degrees' incline. Nothing wrong with this, mind you, but most people will quickly get bored with such repetitive monotony. To jazz things up we offer the following alternatives.

(Source: Walking Magazine December '97 "20 Best Treadmill Workouts")

1. The Retro

The Goal: For coordination, balance and strength.
The Workout: Simply walk backwards on the treadmill at an easy pace.
Total Time: 10-15 minutes.

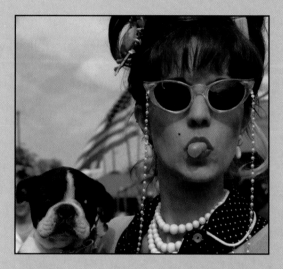

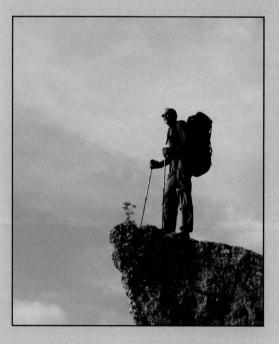

2. The Trail Hike

The Goal: To work a variety of muscle groups (especially your glutes).
The Workout: Use the treadmill's pre-set programs or manually vary the incline while visualizing yourself on a challenging section of the Swiss Alps.
Total Time: 30-45 minutes.

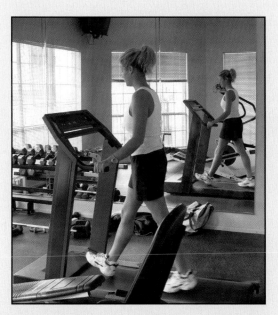

3. The Technique Check

The Goal: To develop efficient walking/running technique.

The Workout: Place mirrors to the front and sides to check your technique – posture, arm swing, and foot action. You can get high-tech and set up a video camera. That's what gait specialists do.

Total Time: 30-60 minutes.

4. The Academy Reward

The Goal: To catch up on classic old movies.

The Workout: Set your treadmill for a comfortable pace and pop in a good walking-related film such as *High Plains Drifter*. If you're a runner try *Chariots of Fire*.

Total Time: Depends on the length of the movie!

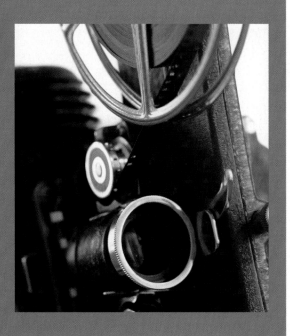

5. Sporting Event "Fartlek"

The Goal: Alternate a very fast pace with a slower pace for quick cardio improvement.
The Workout: Go very quickly during the action on your favorite sport. For example, run during each round of a boxing match, then slow way down during the one-minute breaks.
Total Time: 45-60 minutes

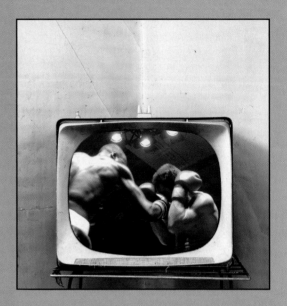

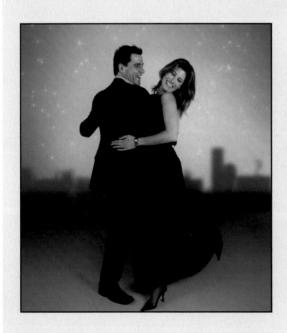

6. The Quick Step

The Goal: To work on foot speed, prevent boredom, and keep occupied during your winter workouts.
The Workout: Count your steps. If you fall below 140 strides per minute, pick up the pace.
Total Time: 45 minutes.

7. The Short Circuit

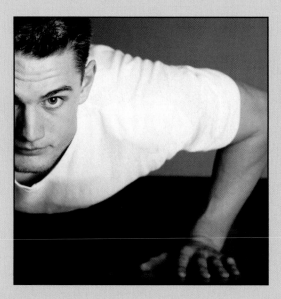

The Goal: A mix of aerobic and strength training.

The Workout: Walk at a comfortable pace for five minutes, then step off and do one minute of circuit exercises. Cycle through crunches, push-ups, lunges and dips. Continue switching back and forth.

Total Time: 30-45 minutes.

8. Rock & Walk

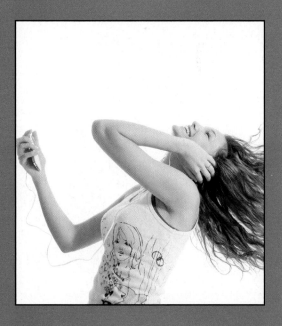

The Goal: Make your workout more fun.

The Workout: Power up the CD or mp3 player while you work out. Try mixing classical, soft rock and hard rock. You can start with soft rock for your warm-up, harder rock or dance music for your workout, then classical or new age for your cool down.

Total Time: Unlimited

9. The Stretch

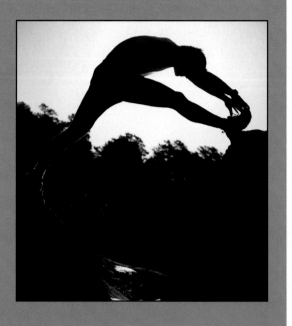

The Goal: A mix of aerobic training and gentle stretching.

The Workout: After an easy 10-minute walk on the treadmill, step off and stretch for five minutes, then continue walking. Every five minutes, slow down and jump off again for one minute to do an easy stretch. Cycle through every major muscle group.

Total Time: 40 minutes.

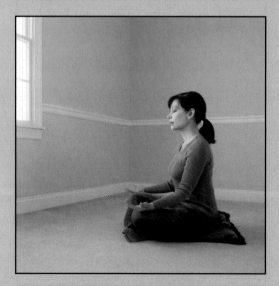

10. Meditation Walk

The Goal: Total relaxation.

The Workout: Light some candles and incense, put on a relaxing new-age music CD and walk your stress away.

Total Time: 30 minutes.

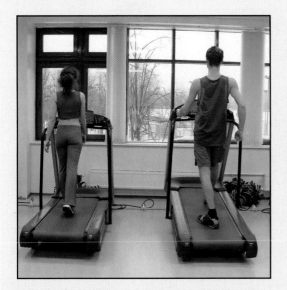

11. The Buddy Walk

The Goal: "Chew the fat" while burning fat.

The Workout: An easy side-by-side walk with your best friend on a pair of treadmills. Nothing makes the time pass like a bit of gossip.

Total Time: 30-60 minutes.

12. The Great Dictator

The Goal: Be "productive" while your creative juices are flowing.

The Workout: Walking workouts are a great time to let the mind wander. Dictate memos, grocery lists, research papers or even the Great American Novel while you walk.

Total Time: 60 minutes.

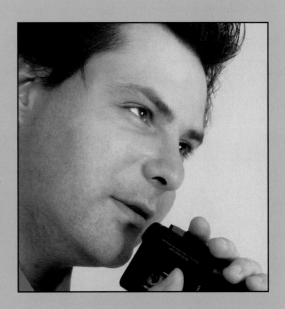

13. Walk Naked

The Goal: The only way to go if you like your workouts "natural".
The Workout: Kinda self-explanatory!
Total Time: As long as you can before you attract an audience.

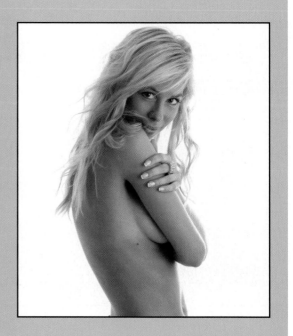

14. Walk to Eat

The Goal: Weight loss.
The Workout: Are those magnets on the refrigerator not working? Instead of useless deterrents, why not "punish" yourself with a 15-minute walk or run on the treadmill every time you open the refrigerator door?
Total Time: 15 minutes (100 - 150 calories) per workout.

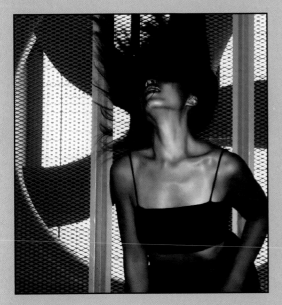

15. The Breeze

The Goal: A refreshing indoor walk.

The Workout: One of the downsides to indoor walks is that the wind doesn't blow through your hair like it does outside. Why not set up a fan a few feet in front of the treadmill for a cool breeze?

Total Time: 45-60 minutes.

16. Pyramid Scheme

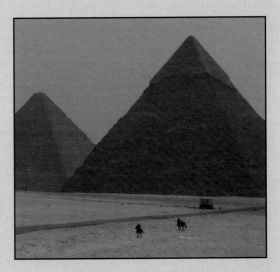

The Goal: A great session for maximum cardiovascular efficiency.

The Workout: After doing an easy 10-minute warm up, do a "pyramid" of fast intervals of 1-2-3-4-5-4-3-2-1 minutes with 2-minute slower-pace "rests" between each fast segment.

Total Time: 40-60 minutes

17. Hill's Afire!

The Goal: Improving your walking technique.

The Workout: Raising the incline to a three- to five-percent grade is the best way to improve your walking technique. The incline forces you to shorten your stride in the front and push more from behind.

Total Time: 20 minutes.

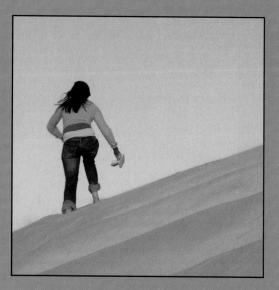

18. Electric Drills

The Goal: Improved technique and interest.

The Workout: After a 10-minute warm-up, break up your walk with 30-second "drill bursts," alternating between long- and short-stride drills. First walk with a very long stride, your arms swinging like pendulums, then walk with a very short stride to practice speed.

Total Time: 30-60 minutes.

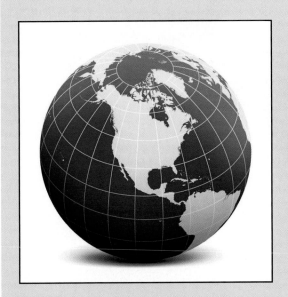

19. The Trans-Continental

The Goal: To circumnavigate the US without leaving your treadmill.
The Workout: Try recording your daily mileage on a wall map with push pins. In no time at all you'll have walked across North America, or even the Earth!
Total Time: Could take years...

20. The Stair Master

The Goal: Great for developing quadriceps strength.
The Workout: If your treadmill's in the basement, this one's for you. Alternate five minutes of treadmill walking with five minutes of walking up and down a flight of stairs.
Total Time: 30 minutes.

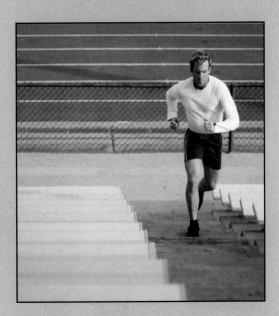

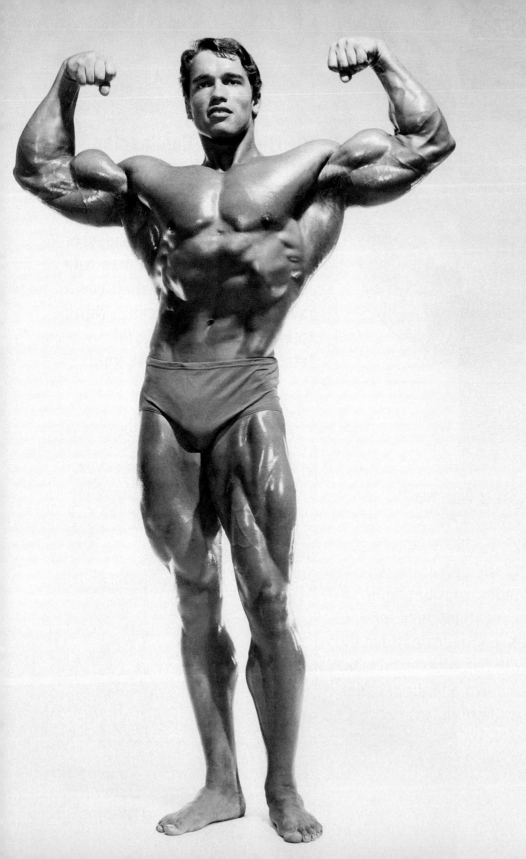

Chapter 4

STRENGTH
TO IMPROVE YOUR
CARDIO

Strength training is a great way to improve your body's shape, improve your functional strength and increase your metabolism, which will help you burn more fat. You can turn to chapter 12 for some good general strength-building exercises. In this chapter I'm just going to give you some exercises specifically to help prepare and condition the body for running and using an elliptical. They don't require any specialized equipment or training apparatus.

Step-Downs

This is a bodyweight exercise. As you develop your strength you may add additional resistance by holding dumbbells.

Technique

Stand on a very stable bench about 18 to 24 inches high. If you are using dumbbells, try to hold them at your sides with a neutral grip (palms facing inwards). Before you start, contract your abdominal muscles to stabilize your torso. Trying to keep most of your weight on one foot, slowly remove the other foot from the bench and step down until your foot is flat on the floor.

Push off the floor and reassume the original standing position on the bench. Repeat the exercise using the other leg. Continue alternating between legs for sets of 10 to 12 reps each.

Tips

• Don't hold your breath. Exhale on the downward portion and inhale on the upward portion.

• Keep good posture, with your back in a vertical position.

• Do not allow the knee of the forward leg to extend past the toes of the foot.

• Never lock your knees at any point during this exercise.

• The downward portion of this exercise should be performed slowly and with full control.

Bench Step-Ups

This is another body-weight exercise that can be modified by holding on to dumbbells.

Technique

Stand in an upright position and contract your abdominal muscles to stabilize your trunk and spine. Stand directly in front of and facing the bench and place one foot (lead foot) flat on the bench. With most of your weight on the heel of the lead foot, forcefully push off with the lead leg and assume a standing position, with both feet on the bench. Slowly remove the trailing leg from the bench and lower yourself to the original starting position. Repeat this exercise using the other leg as the lead leg.

Tips

• Don't hold your breath. Exhale on the downward movement and inhale on the upward.

• Keep good posture, with your back in a vertical position.

• Do not allow the knee of the forward leg to extend past the toes of the foot.

• Never lock your knees at any point during this exercise.

• The downward portion of this exercise should be performed

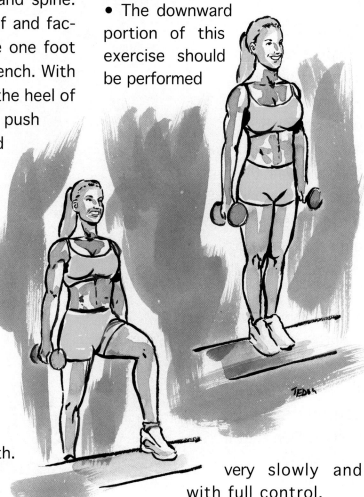

very slowly and with full control.

Dumbbell Arm Swing

This exercise is performed using light dumbbells, or you could even hold cans of vegetables or soup, as long as you have a good grip on them.

Technique

Adopt a runner's stance, with one leg in front and one behind. Hold a light dumbbell in each hand and, with the arms bent at the elbows, forcefully swing your arms as you would when running.

Tips

• All the movement should be at the shoulder joint.

• Always keep control of the weight. Don't let it control you.

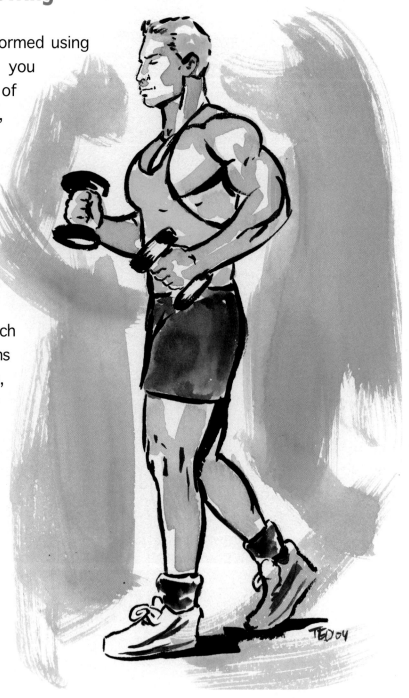

One-Leg Squats

This is a body-weight exercise. Those with strong legs can increase the resistance by holding dumbbells.

Technique

Stand in an upright position and contract your abdominal muscles to stabilize the trunk and spine. Place one foot (rear foot) behind you on a bench that is about one foot high (you can use the bottom step on a set of stairs if need be). Your other foot (forward foot) should be flat on the floor and directly under you. Slowly bend your forward knee until your thigh is parallel with the floor. Try not to let your knee extend in front of your toes. Slowly straighten your forward leg and return to the starting upright position. Repeat using the other leg.

Tips

• Don't hold your breath. Exhale on the downward movement and inhale on the upward.

• Keep good posture, with your back in a vertical position throughout the movement.

• Do not allow the knee of the forward leg to extend past the toes.

• Never lock your knees at any point during this exercise.

• The downward portion of this exercise should be performed very slowly and with full control.

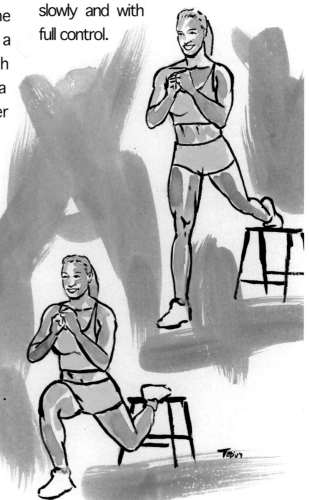

Lunge With Medicine Ball

Take a long step forward with one leg, keeping the knee and foot of the forward leg aligned. Slowly bend the knee of the forward leg until the thigh is parallel to the floor. At the same time lower the knee of the trailing leg toward the floor. The knee of the rear leg should stop approximately two inches from the floor. Always try to keep your upper body in a vertical position.

Repeat this exercise with the legs in opposite positions.

Tips

• Don't hold your breath. Exhale on the downward portions and inhale on the upward portion.

• Keep good posture with your back in a vertical position.

• Do not allow the knee of the forward leg to extend past the toes.

• Never lock your knees at any point during this exercise.

• The downward portion of this exercise should be performed very slowly and with full control.

If you don't have access to a medicine ball, you can perform this as a bodyweight exercise.

Technique

This exercise is performed with a medicine ball.

Stand in an upright position and hold the medicine ball in front of you. Contract your abdominal muscles to stabilize your trunk and spine.

Side Lunge

This is a body-weight exercise.

Technique

As with the previous exercises, this exercise may be performed with body weight or with additional resistance by holding dumbbells. Stand in an upright position and contract your abdominal muscles to stabilize your trunk and spine. Take a long step sideways with one leg. Keep the knee and foot of the moving leg aligned. Slowly bend the side-moving knee until the thigh is parallel to the floor. At the same time, lower the knee of the trailing leg towards the floor. The trailing leg should remain straight. With your upper body held in a vertical position, forcefully push off with the side leg and bring it back into position with the trailing leg. You should now be back in the starting position. Repeat for the other leg.

Tips

• Don't hold your breath. Exhale on the downward movement and inhale on the upward.

• Keep good posture, with your back in a vertical position.

• Do not allow the knee of the forward leg to extend past the toes.

• Never lock your knees at any point during this exercise.

• The downward portion of this exercise should be performed very slowly and with full control.

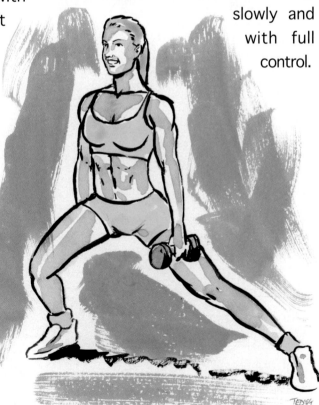

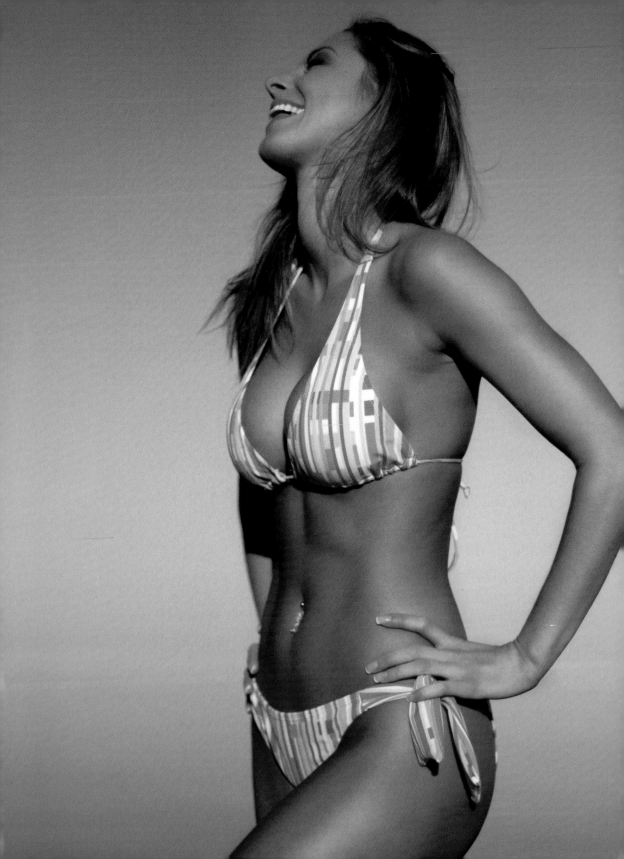

Chapter 6

STAY MOTIVATED

If getting down on your hands and knees and cleaning the toilet with a toothbrush seems like more fun than doing your workout, it's time to rethink your relationship with your machine. If you feel yourself starting to slip into this way of thinking, change your attitude. Follow these tips to keep you and your machine on speaking terms.

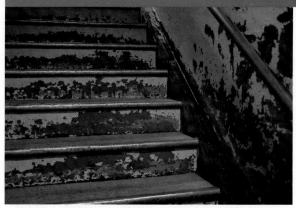

Where would you prefer to work out?

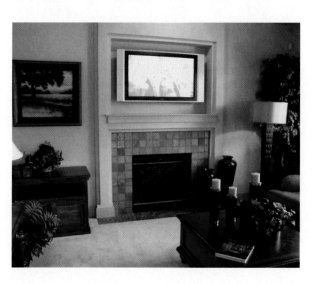

Mood swings.

Put your treadmill in an inviting place so you have easy access to entertainment like your TV, CD player or radio. Get it out of that cold, dark basement. Even the most dedicated of exercisers would have trouble getting motivated in such a depressing environment.

If the gym is your preferred location for using the treadmill, take advantage of the many entertainment options at your disposal. If your gym's entertainment system doesn't appeal to you, bring your own. **A portable CD player or iPod is a great fitness investment.** Stock it up with your favourite tunes and start running.

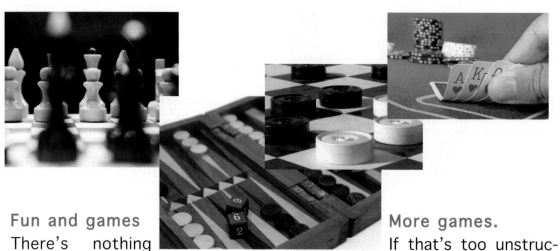

Fun and games

There's nothing like a few mind games to carry you through a run or power walk. Say to yourself: "For the next three minutes I'm going to run at 5 mph, then I'll walk for three minutes at 3.5 mph. Then I'll run at 7 mph for two minutes before walking for another three minutes. Keep this up until your workout is complete.

More games.

If that's too unstructured for you, come up with a definite plan beforehand. For example, try a pyramid. Increase your speed 0.1 mph every minute until you hit the halfway point of your workout, say 15 minutes. Then for the next 15 minutes decrease the speed 0.1 mph every minute.

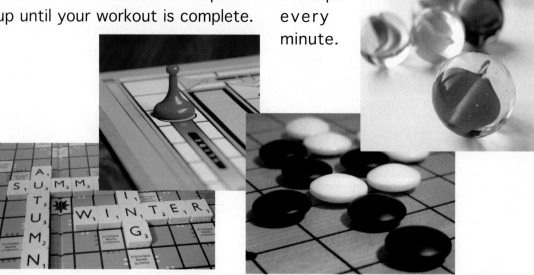

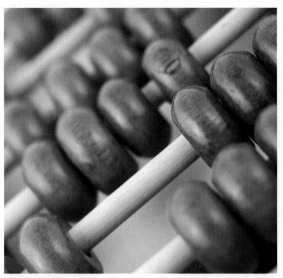

Counting steps

Similar to "Fun and Games," counting steps involves switching your incline or speed, but you do it with a number of steps ... try 100. So you might walk for 100 steps, run for 100 steps, put the incline to 8 percent for 100 steps, etc. One hundred steps is not very much, so it's easy to convince yourself to keep going.

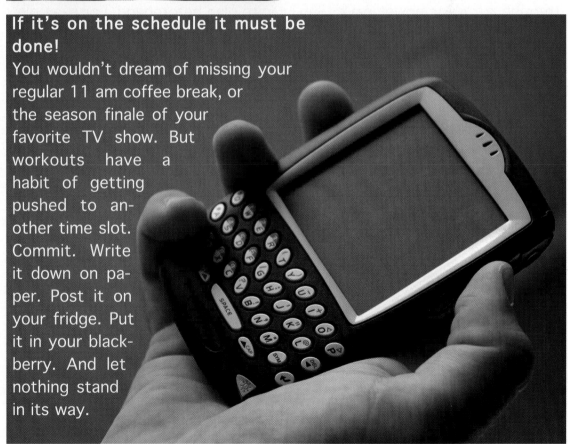

If it's on the schedule it must be done!

You wouldn't dream of missing your regular 11 am coffee break, or the season finale of your favorite TV show. But workouts have a habit of getting pushed to another time slot. Commit. Write it down on paper. Post it on your fridge. Put it in your blackberry. And let nothing stand in its way.

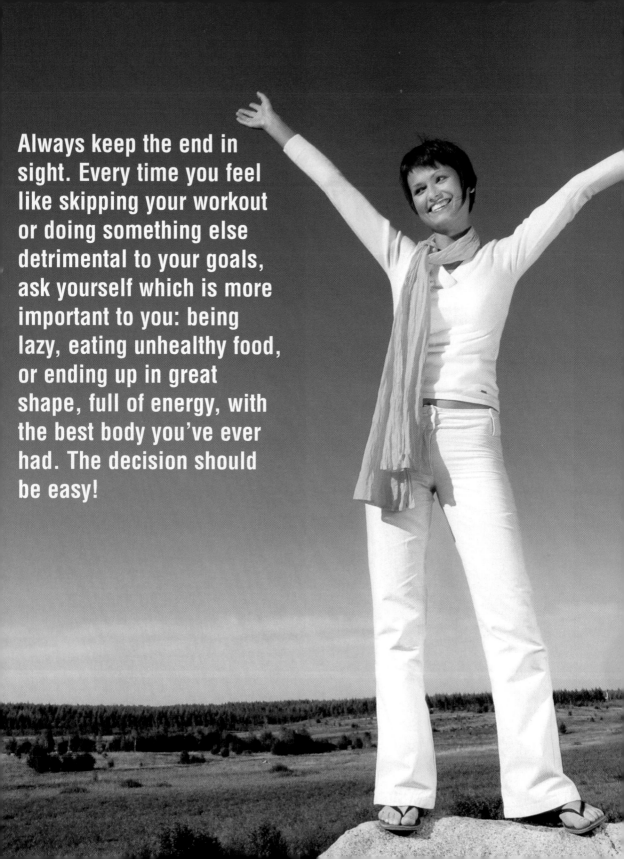

Always keep the end in sight. Every time you feel like skipping your workout or doing something else detrimental to your goals, ask yourself which is more important to you: being lazy, eating unhealthy food, or ending up in great shape, full of energy, with the best body you've ever had. The decision should be easy!

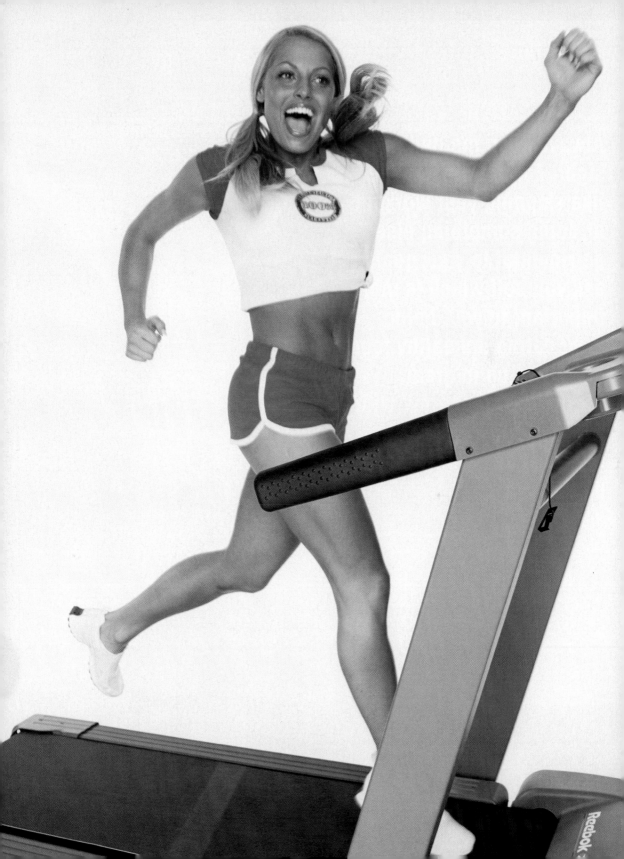

Chapter 7

TRISH STRATUS AND HER

TREADMILL WORKOUT

Trish's Fitness Beginnings

Her beauty is second to none, and her brains and brawn make her the total feminine package. She started out as a fitness model, then Trish Stratus entered the WWE (World Wrestling Entertainment) in 2000, first as a manager for several

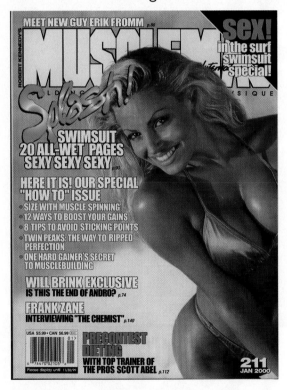

young superstars. However, her beauty and athleticism left the fans asking for more, so Trish worked her way to the top of the WWE Women's Division. Trish, who recently retired from wrestling, held the WWE Women's Championship title on several occasions and was always in the mix to challenge for the top spot and headline a major WWE event.

Many assume that Trish's great physique is the result of having the right parents. While she is first to admit that she had a few advantages in the gene pool, **she has had to work extremely hard to perfect her physique.**

Trish's road to physical perfection started when she was introduced to noted Canadian trainer, Scott Abel. Scott immediately recognized Trish's great potential and took her to the offices of *MuscleMag International* to meet Robert Kennedy. Bob has always had a reputation for spotting talent, and it took only one test shoot to realize that Trish had that something special.

Under Scott's experienced training eye, Trish continued to make great improvements to her physique, and it wasn't long before she was gracing the covers of fitness magazines and books. From covers and books, Trish rapidly progressed to radio and TV talk shows and the rest, as they say, is history.

Trish's Leg- and Butt-Training Strategy

When Trish first started training, her lower body overpowered her upper body. She attributes this to her high school soccer and field hockey days. The many miles of running during practice and games gave her legs and glutes a great foundation to improve upon. But when Trish got into serious training, both she and Scott realized her legs and glutes had a few pounds of fat that she could do without.

Unlike many women who are afraid to use weights for fear of "looking like Arnold," **Trish realized that nothing shapes a woman's body like weight training does.** She has therefore made strength training a staple part of her exercise program.

Because of her hectic schedule and lack of free time, Trish has devised a series of training routines that are quick but highly effective. She uses at least 20 reps for lower body exercises, and utilizes numerous intensity-increasing methods to get more accomplished in less time, such as supersets (alternating two exercises before rest), trisets (alternating three exercises), and giant sets (alternating four or more exercises).

During a hectic stretch of WWE scheduling **Trish normally gets in two to three weight-training workouts a week.** If she has more time, however, she splits her body into six parts and does one part each day, training six days per week.

Trish's Unique Treadmill Workout

Since she's always on the go, Trish has had to be creative when it comes to working her body, especially her legs and butt. When she first started traveling with the WWE, Trish discovered that many of the smaller towns had primitive training conditions. **Since the one piece of equipment that virtually all gyms and hotels have is the treadmill, she began to use it** creatively as the mainstay of her workouts.

When she first began doing her unique lunges and one-leg squats on treadmills, Trish garnered many strange looks and comments. But as soon as anyone tried the workout, he or she quickly discovered that Trish was onto something.

Trish starts her treadmill workout by walking for two minutes to warm up both her muscles and cardio system. She keeps the speed at a comfortable walking pace and the incline at zero. She then slows the speed down to about 1.5 miles per hour to start the real work. Her first activity is one-leg calf raises. While walking she focuses her weight on her front foot and rises up on her toes to perform calf raises. Her legs are scissored, and as the front heel rises off the ground to contract the calf muscle, the back heel stays down, providing a good stretch.

Figure 1

After her calf work, Trish switches to lunges (figure 1) for 20 reps per leg. Next are one-legged squats, working the front leg with the back leg straight. Again she'll do 15 to 20 reps per side. By this point her thighs and glutes are burning, so she does the calf raises again to give them a rest. Back to her thighs, she does a move she calls "pushing a baby carriage," which is similar to a very long-stride lunge (figure 2). Trish usually rotates the exercises for 30 to 45 minutes.

Although this is Trish's typical treadmill workout, she's been known to change things up. Sometimes she'll do her treadmill routine after her weight-training workout – even a hard one. Trish also makes frequent use of dumbbells during her treadmill training, doing such exercises as biceps curls, kickbacks, flyes, and lateral raises. In addition, she does various swinging and punching motions, making sure she works out her entire body, especially if she doesn't have access to a full gym.

Great legs and buns don't just magically appear. You have to work hard to give them that knockout look. By combining a good diet with regular cardio and strength training, you can build the lower body that you always dreamed about. You can't go wrong in adopting Trish Stratus' treadmill workout.

Figure 2

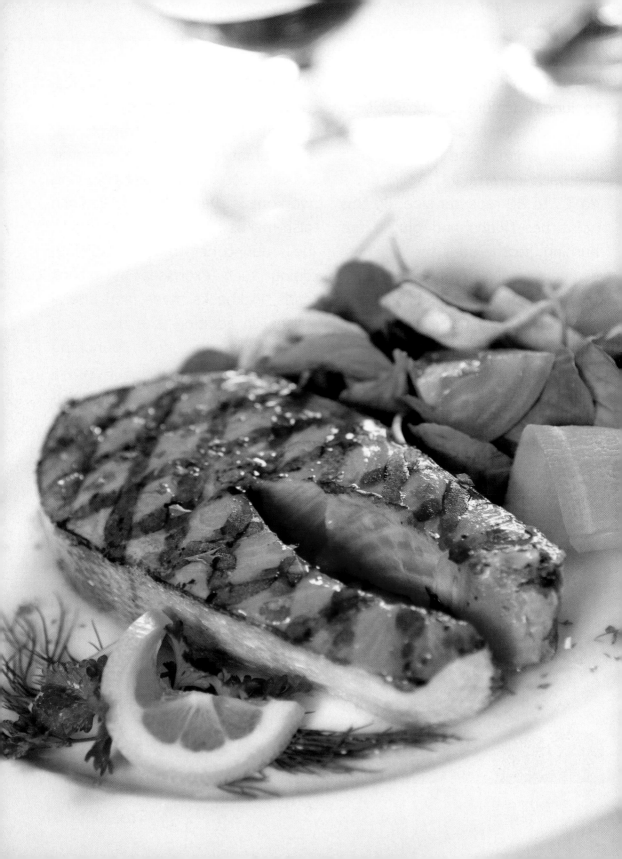

Chapter 8

NUTRITION FOR A GREAT BODY

The Key

If not the most important aspect to getting the body you want, your diet is certainly one of the most important aspects. You have to eat good food to look good. But those who want to look great have to go that extra mile and eat great!

You're probably sick and tired of hearing it but it's true; a balanced diet is the key to ultimate nutrition and health.

However, **eating a great diet is not always that easy.** Many people feel that they're too busy to eat properly. It's often easier to eat junk food than to take a few extra minutes and prepare a healthy meal. **The problem with fast food is that it can lead to a fast death!** Most grease joints serve nothing but food that is high in fat – especially trans fat – and calories and low in other nutrients. This can seriously affect your health. At the other extreme, there is a multi-billion dollar industry focused on telling women that being fit means being ultra-thin and that starving yourself is part of good nutrition.

When you combine busy lives with social propaganda, it's no wonder that many women suffer from poor eating habits. **Good nutrition means eating a balanced diet.** It's important to learn how to eat right, and this means eating the right amounts of the right kinds of food.

In theory nutritious eating isn't that difficult. In fact most readers

probably know the basics. You should be consuming a diet that includes plenty of fruits and vegetables, whole-grain products, fish, chicken, and lean red meat. Your intake of saturated fats, sugar and salt should be restricted. Even something as simple as getting enough water is important; you should drink at least eight, 8-ounce glasses of water daily (more if you exercise frequently).

Don't Skip Meals!

If you regularly skip breakfast and eat a small lunch, you'll be ravenous later in the day. It may seem counterintuitive, but **most people who skip meals eat more calories per day than those who do not.**

However, there is another reason skipping meals will keep you fat. **Whenever you skip a meal, your body slows down its metabolism and begins releasing calorie-storing hormones.** Your

body doesn't realize that you have a nice big dinner waiting for you later. As far as it knows you may have to wait days before eating again, and its goal is to stay alive, not to be thin.

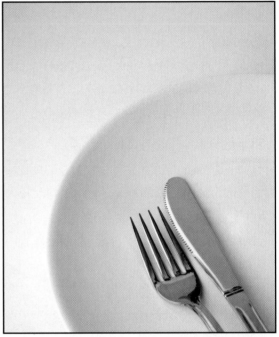

The best way to combat this phenomenon is by eating smaller meals frequently. Spread these small meals throughout the day. This not only keeps your metabolism revved up, but also tricks the body into not slipping into any type of calorie (and fat) conserving mode.

The Digestive System – The Incredible Journey

Every time food passes your lips, it marks the beginning of an incredible journey.

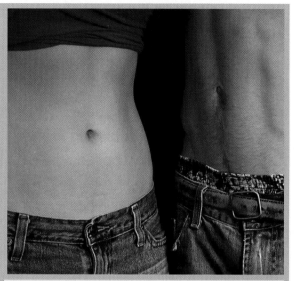

Stage 1 – The Mouth

The instant food enters your mouth your digestive system kicks in. The taste buds come alive and start transmitting messages to your brain so you can distinguish between sweet, salty, bitter, and sour sensations.

While your taste buds are doing their thing, your teeth are grinding food down into smaller, more easily digested piec-es. Saliva is added to moisten everything so that it doesn't tear your digestive (gastrointestinal) tract on the way down. In addition, the saliva itself helps to break your food down.

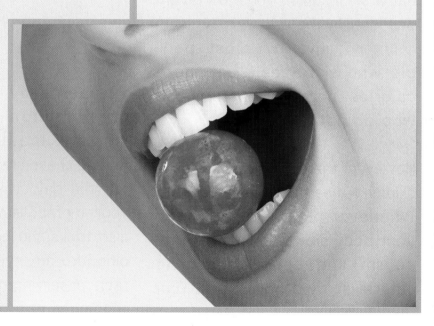

Stage 2 – The Stomach

Once swallowed, the food is carried down the esophagus to the second-site digestion - the stomach. Your stomach walls churn the food up to make sure that it's mixed with your acidic digestive juices. By the time food leaves the stomach, it is a creamy mixture called chyme (pronounced kime). Once in this liquid state it can easily travel to the small intestine.

Once the food has been broken down into tiny particles, much of it is absorbed through the walls of your small intestine and the nutrients are carried into your blood-

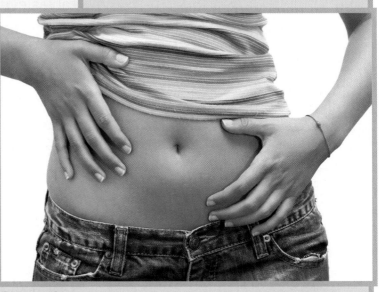

Stage 3 – The Small Intestine

Most of the nutrient-digesting action happens in the small intestine. To help your small intestine cope with the acidity of the partially digested food, your pancreas releases lots of alkaline (basic) enzymes, which serve to further break down protein, fat, and carbohydrate. Your gall bladder releases bile, to ensure that fat is given a thorough going over.

stream. The average adult has between 20 and 24 feet of small intestine stacked throughout his or her lower abdomen.

Stage 4 – The Large Intestine

To cope with more difficult nutrients, the body has a fourth site of digestion called the large intestine. For example, fiber is a nutrient with certain components that can't be absorbed by the human body.

Your large intestine acts like a storage and processing tank to break down fiber and other tough food products. Besides digestive juices, the large intestine gets help from bacteria, which do wonders with dense plant material. Whatever the large intestine can't handle becomes waste matter and is stored in the rectum for release at the most convenient opportunity.

The Food Groups

Fruit and Vegetables

Numerous scientific studies have shown that people who regularly include plenty of fruit and vegetables in their diets are at lower risk of developing illnesses such as heart disease and some cancers. For this reason health authorities recommend that you eat at least five, and preferably ten, servings of fruit and vegetables every day. And while raw, fresh vegetables and fruit are generally best for you, frozen, cooked, dried, and even tinned are certainly better than not eating them at all. **Aim for at least one portion of fruit or vegetables at every meal.**

The next time you're shopping, toss a few new fruits or vegetables into your basket – either something that you've never tried before or something you turned your nose up at as a child. Tastes change over time. If you experiment, you'll give your mouth a treat and do your body a favor.

Don't be Colorblind

If you're worried about whether you're getting the right amount of nutrients from your fruits and vegetables, try adding a bit of color. Many nutritionists recommend choosing your fruits and vegetables based on color. Eat something green, something red, and something yellow or orange at least once a day to guarantee a good mix of vitamins and minerals in your diet.

Keep in mind that it is far better to get your fruit servings from eating fruit than it is from drinking juice, especially if you're trying to lose weight. One four-ounce glass of orange juice has the same calories as an entire orange, with none of the fiber. But who drinks four ounces? Most glasses of juice are about 12 ounces of refined fructose.

How can you fit all these fruits and vegetables into your life? Easy!

Breakfast: One glass of orange or grapefruit juice (1)
plus
Oatmeal or cold cereal with sliced banana and berries (1)

Snack:
Protein shake with banana or berries blended in (1)

Lunch:
Vegetable soup (1)
Side salad (1)

Dinner:
One cup mixed vegetables (1)
One-half baked sweet potato (1)

Dessert or snack:
Fresh strawberries with yogurt. (1)

There you go, eight servings.
That wasn't so hard, now, was it?

Milk and Dairy Products

This oft-maligned food group includes milk, cheese, yogurt, butter, margarine and cream. The foods in this group contain many different kinds of nutrients, but they're particularly rich in calcium. They can also be high in fat, so you must choose items from this group with discretion.

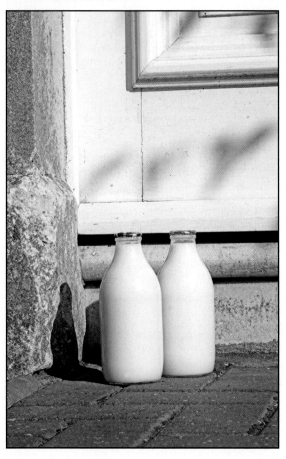

The Importance of Calcium

Calcium is a major component of bones and teeth. It is also involved in muscle contraction and conduction of electricity through your nervous system. It is especially important for growth, and this important mineral will continue to be added to your bones until you reach your mid 30s. After this point, **the natural aging process begins to leech calcium from the bones, causing them to lose their strength and density,** possibly leading to osteoporosis.

Health professionals estimate that **one in three women and one in ten men will develop severe osteoporosis** at some point in their lives, and there's concern that teenage girls and young women are at particular risk, given their preoccupation with fad diets. Many of these diets are calcium deficient and some experts predict that a whole generation of women could be at risk for developing osteoporosis earlier in life.

Calcium and the Vegetarian or Lactose Intolerant

Those who follow strict vegetarian diets and exclude milk products from their diets or those who can't tolerate the milk sugar called lactose need to look for calcium alternatives. You can still keep your bones healthy by buying dairy products made with soy that have been enriched with calcium. Don't forget that dark green leafy vegetables such as spinach and broccoli are high in calcium.

How Much Calcium?

The US Department of Health recommends that men and women who are not pregnant or nursing get approximately 700 to 800 mg of calcium every day to ensure good health. In terms of servings this means:

• One pint of milk
• Two small yogurt containers
• About 80 g of hard cheese

From a weight loss or weight maintenance point of view the good news is that you can get all the calcium you need while avoiding full-fat foods. Skimmed milk contains exactly the same amount of calcium as whole milk. Only the fat

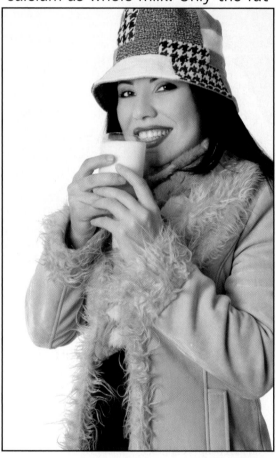

has been removed, not the mineral. The same goes for low-fat yogurt and cheese; you don't have to buy their high-fat relatives to keep your bones strong and healthy.

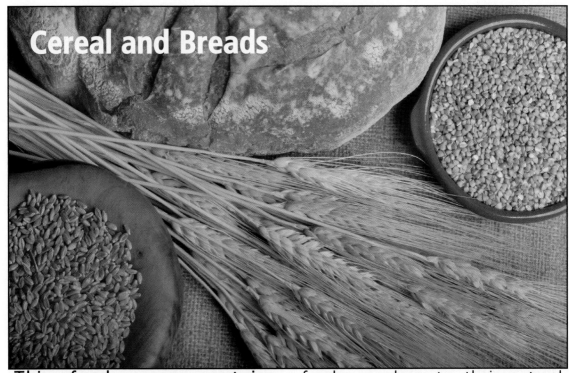

Cereal and Breads

This food group contains pasta, rice, breads, grains, and cereals. This group is high in complex carbohydrates and starch – your body's main sources of energy.

Refined and Unrefined Carbohydrates

Most of the foods listed in this group began life as grains, including rice, barley, wheat, corn, and rye. Grains are very healthy and filling, but you should eat these foods as close to their natural state as possible. Always choose whole-grain versions.

Refined carbohydrates are those for which machinery has been used to remove the high-fiber components from the grain. White bread, white rice, sugary cereals, and most pasta (made from white flour) are all examples of refined carbohydrates. While food companies may tell you that their cereal "contains

12 essential nutrients and is a part of a healthy breakfast," in reality this refining process creates nutrient-deficient food.

Unrefined carbohydrates, on the other hand, contain the whole grain. They contain their full complement of vitamins and minerals. They're higher in fiber and will keep you feeling fuller for longer periods of time. This tends to reduce your food consumption; important if you're trying to lose weight and don't like hunger pangs. Some examples are brown rice, whole-wheat bread, oats, and whole-wheat pastas. It should be said here that we consume far too much bread. Although whole-wheat bread is certainly better than white, any flour is refined and should be eaten sparingly.

Simple and complex carbohydrates

These two terms are often confused with refined and unrefined, but really refer to the chemical structure of the carbohydrate molecule rather than to whether the grain is whole. Complex carbohydrates are more difficult for the body to break down, because their structure is, well, complex! Therefore **they provide you with nutrients over an extended period of time, helping to regulate blood sugar.** Most natural forms of carbohydrates are indeed complex, with the exception of fruit. Although fruit contains simple sugars, it also contains fiber, which helps combat the fact that it breaks down quickly. Keep in mind that this is the case when fruit is eaten whole. Fruit consumed as juice is missing that fiber. Be careful not to go overboard on fruit juice, it can really cause you to pack on the pounds.

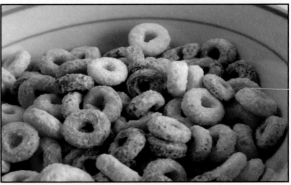

Starch

Contrary to popular belief, starches are not fattening. What usually makes starch "fattening" is all the high-fat sauces, oils, and creams, often added to otherwise healthy rice and potatoes. Even pastas and breads can be enoyed in moderation, and as long as they are made with whole grains.

Fiber

Fiber doesn't supply much in the way of nutrients but is vital in helping your body process waste efficiently. In addition, fiber helps you to feel full for longer periods of time, helping you to eat less.

Glycogen

Glycogen is the body's storage form of simple sugar. It's primarily formed from glucose, and serves as the body's chief form of energy.

How Much is Enough?

Most nutritionists recommend that the bulk of your diet - roughly 50 percent - should come from carbohydrates. You should also get at least 20 grams of fiber a day. An easy way to ensure that you get enough is to include a representative from this food at every meal. **Try to eat only fiber-rich, unrefined carbohydrates.** Here are a few healthy suggestions:

- **Oatmeal with yogurt, raisins and berries for breakfast**

- **Sandwich made with whole-wheat bread for lunch**

- **Seafood with vegetables and brown rice for supper**

- **Plenty of vegetables at mealtime and fresh fruit for snacks.**

Meat, Poultry, Fish and Other Protein Sources

Besides meat products, you can include, nuts, beans, seeds, soya products, and vegetable protein.

The Highs and Lows of Protein

Protein plays an essential role in the building and repairing of your body's various organs and tissues. But whether a particular molecule helps your hair grow or repairs an exercised muscle depends very much on what the protein is composed of. This is because protein is made up of smaller units called polypeptide chains, which in turn are composed of amino acids. The unique sequence of these 22 amino acids gives the protein its unique characteristics.

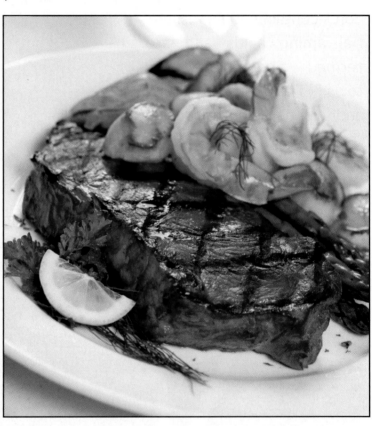

Some amino acids can be manufactured by your body, and are called nonessential amino acids. The eight amino acids that cannot be manufactured are called essential amino acids. These must be consumed through food. **Though all animal and plant cells contain protein, there is a wide difference in the quantity and quality.**

Complete and Incomplete

Foods such as meat, fish, poultry, eggs, and milk are called "complete proteins" because they contain all the essential amino acids. On the other hand, most plant sources don't contain enough essential amino acids and are termed "incomplete proteins." The exceptions are soy and quinoa – both considered "superfoods" because of their superior nutritional composition.

While beans and other vegetarian choices contain protein, these sources do not contain all the essential amino acids. If the body does not receive all of the essential amino acids at one time, it begins leaching its own muscle for those that are missing. This means that vegetarians need to do some clever protein combining at meals to ensure that the amino acid of one incomplete protein can compensate for the deficiencies of another.

The egg is such a good source of protein that all other sources are measured against it.

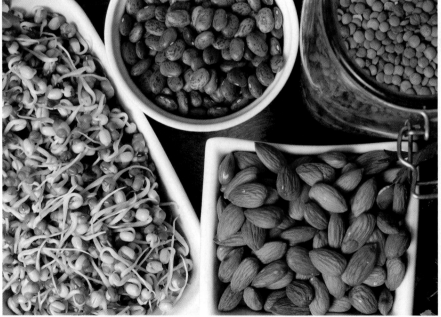

Fats and Oils

Because of its high calorie density, fat has gotten such a bad rap that many people try to avoid it entirely. Yet fat is actually an important contributor to optimum health. You just have to be careful to choose the right *kinds* of fat.

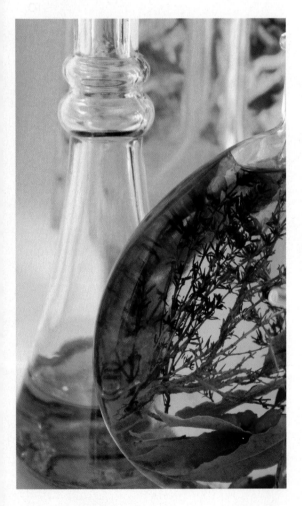

Fat Facts

Despite the amount of negative press it has received over the years, fat is a vital nutrient and plays a role in such biological processes as:

• transporting fat-soluble vitmins A, D, E and K throughout the body.

• cushioning and protecting internal organs.

• keeping skin, hair and nails healthy.

• making food taste better, and giving it a better texture.

• believe it or not, some fats help you control your body-fat level.

Essential fatty acids (EFAs) are necessary for the proper functioning of your cardiovascular, endocrine, and immune systems, and fat is a concentrated source of energy. When you think about it, it's astonishing how our bodies are ready for almost any condition, including starvation – which it seeks to avoid by storing energy for later use. Our bodies

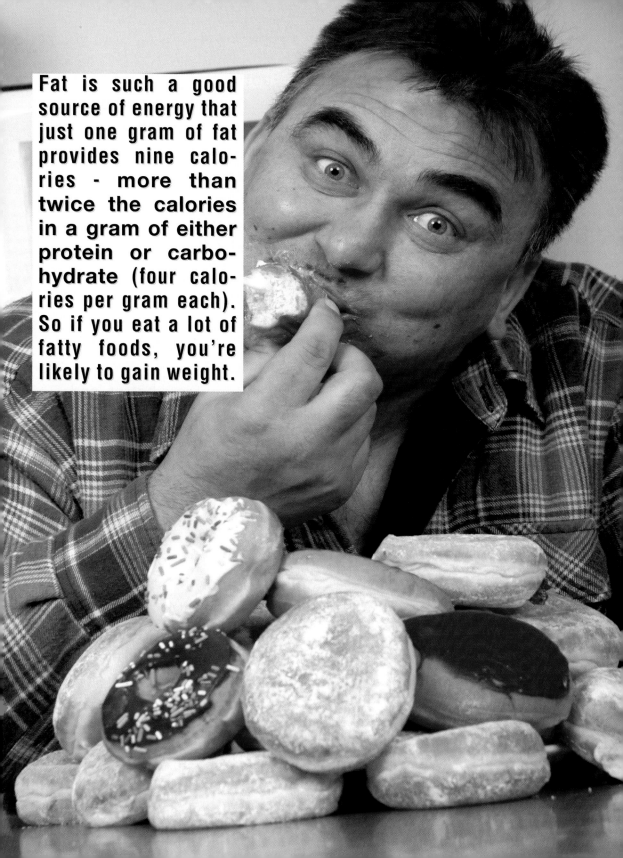

Fat is such a good source of energy that just one gram of fat provides nine calories - more than twice the calories in a gram of either protein or carbohydrate (four calories per gram each). So if you eat a lot of fatty foods, you're likely to gain weight.

just don't seem to understand that we have enough food these days in this country ... in fact, we have more than enough!

● ●

Not all fat is created equal. Fat comes in two main forms and there is a world of difference between the two.

Saturated and Unsaturated

When we think of artery-clogging, health-destroying fat we are really thinking about saturated fat. **Saturated fat is generally solid at room temperature and it's usually derived from animal sources.** It's the fat in such foods as butter, cheese, and whole milk. It's also the white fat you see on red meat and underneath chicken skin. The less saturated fat you eat, the better. No exceptions. Few things in nutrition are absolutely certain but a high intake of saturated fat is almost guaranteed to lead to coronary heart disease.

Trans fat is a type of saturated fat, but it's a particularly bad type. Trans fat is created when hydrogen is added to an unsaturated fat. This is done for two reasons: to prevent separation, as in margarine or processed peanut butter, and to create good "mouthfeel," a term used by food manufacturers to describe a pleasant feeling the consumer experiences when he or she eats the product.

Just a couple of years ago people thought that products made with hydrogenated vegetable oils were better for you than saturated fat. That has now been proven false. In fact, **trans fats are so bad for you that lobby groups are trying to make them illegal.** Because of a loophole in new labelling laws some products even proudly proclaim themselves to be trans-fat free when in fact they are not. Read food labels. *Avoid any food item that contains partially hydrogenated or hydrogenated oils.*

Unsaturated fat is liquid at room temperature. It usually comes from vegetable sources, though many types of fish are rich sources. The two types of unsaturated fat are monounsaturated and polyunsaturated. Both types are far healthier than saturated fat, but many consider monounsaturated to be the best. The best sources are nuts and seeds, olive oil, sunflower, soya and canola oils, and such deep-water fish as mackerel, sardines, herring, and salmon.

How Much is Enough?

Government guidelines recommend that fat make up no more than 35 percent of your diet. In fact this is definitely on the generous side. Try keeping your fat intake to 20 to 25 percent of your diet.

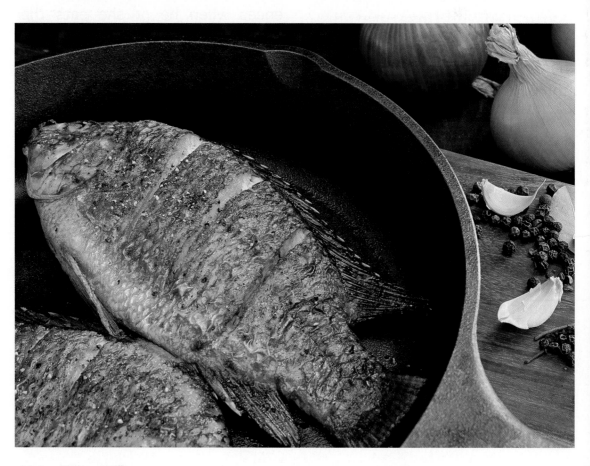

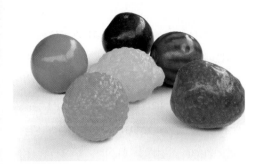

Sugary Foods

Like fat, sugar is a concentrated source of energy and has also developed a bad reputation over the years. **Although we need fat in our diet, we definitely do not need sugar.** Be that as it may, high-sugar foods such as cookies, candies, chocolate and soft drinks have become ingrained in our nutritional consciousness. They taste great and we consider them treats.

Despite the psychological boost to our pallet, high-sugar foods can play havoc with our health, and everything from diabetes to tooth decay to obesity and cardiovascular disease is amplified by excessive sugar intake. The occasional cookie or small dessert is fine, but try to make it a once-a-week treat, not an everyday occurrence.

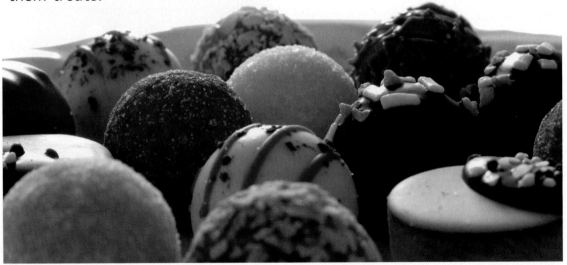

Snacking

Most nutritionists will admit that snacking regularly throughout the day is good for you. However, **some types of snacks you *should* be consuming,** and some you definitely shouldn't! There's a huge difference between eating potato chips and eating an apple.

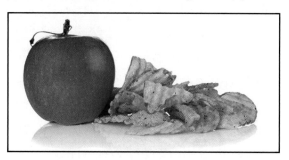

Surveys show that over 95 percent of North Americans snack at least once a day. Unfortunately they generally snack on foods that contain high amounts of fat, sugar and cholesterol. Many people consume more calories in their snacks than they do in their meals.

Choosing healthy foods for snacks is just as important as deciding what to eat for your regular meals.

Healthy snacks can add extra nutrients and fiber to your diet without unwanted calories. They'll give you an energy boost during the day, keep your metabolism running high, and help you cut down on overeating at your regular meals.

Instead of that chocolate bar or bag of chips, reach for an orange, pear, or some cherry tomatoes. For about 50 calories you'll get

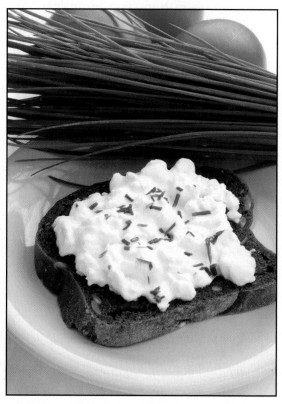

extra fiber, vitamins, and minerals. **Add some yogurt, cottage cheese, a boiled egg or some low-fat cheese and you've done a great deal to aid in your weight loss and your sugar and metabolic regulation.**

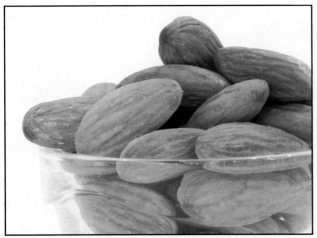

Nuts, too (especially raw almonds) are a great snack. You don't want to have more than a handful, because they do have a high fat content. But please **don't let their high fat content scare you away.** They have a host of important vitamins and minerals, and the fat they contain is the very best kind – the omegas, which actually work to lower bad cholesterol and raise good cholesterol.

If you keep your food portions small and space your meals and snacks two to three hours apart, you won't gain weight. Also, keep your snacks under 250 calories. Food labels will help you calculate the number of calories in foods by portion size, but please pay attention to the portion size stated on the package. **Many companies are deceitful with regard to portion sizes to make it look as if their products contain fewer calories than they actually do.**

Nutrition Facts

Servings Per Container 8

Amount Per Serving

Calories 200   Calories from Fat 45

% Daily Value*

Total Fat 5g   8%

Saturated Fat 2.5g

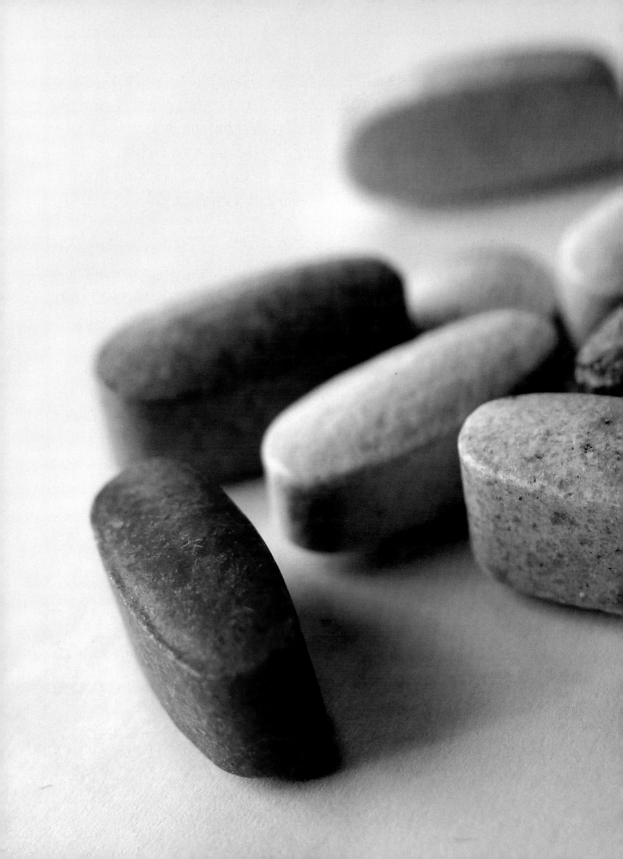

Chapter 9

SUPPLEMENTS

Supplements

The shelves of health food stores are loaded with an alphabet of vitamins and supplements these days. **Every week seems to bring some new product** that will revitalize you, increase your longevity or improve your immune system. Understandably, the prevailing questions that most people have are "do I need to use any of them, and if so, which ones?"

Be wary of marketing claims. Many products out there rely more on hype than on legitimate science. Some could even be harmful. To be honest, the best supplements are in the produce aisle of your local supermarket! You'll also be ingesting numerous cancer-preventing phytochemicals and other helpful natural compounds that science can't put into a bottle. That said, there are occasions when supplements are a good idea.

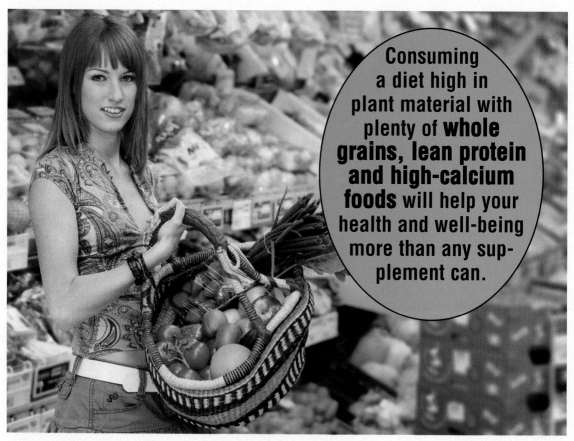

Consuming a diet high in plant material with plenty of **whole grains, lean protein and high-calcium foods** will help your health and well-being more than any supplement can.

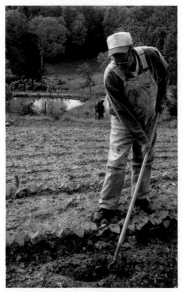

• Everyone should take a multivitamin/mineral supplement. Modern farming practices have severely depleted the vitamins and minerals offered by food. **Unless you grow all your own food in humus-rich soil and raise all your meat naturally, then taking a multivitamin/mineral daily is a good idea.**

• If you don't get enough calcium from dairy products and leafy green vegetables, **consider taking a calcium supplement.** As with most supplements, you can increase the benefit by taking smaller amounts throughout the day rather than a lot all at once, to improve absorption. In addition, calcium works in conjunction with magnesium, so take a supplement that contains both minerals. (As a bonus, Cal-Mag tablets can be used both as a sleeping aid and to help get rid of headaches.)

• **Those who exercise heavily sometimes need a little more than diet can offer.** For example, those who do heavy weight training or sprinting need more protein than the average person, and may have a difficult time consuming that much through diet alone.

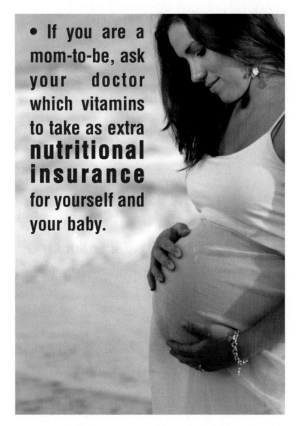

• **If you are a mom-to-be, ask your doctor which vitamins to take as extra nutritional insurance for yourself and your baby.**

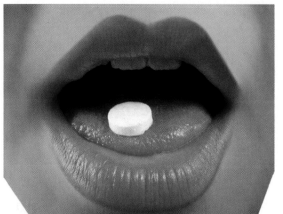

Choose supplements from major manufacturers. Keep in mind that the industry is poorly regulated and you may not be getting the quantity or quality of nutrient listed on the label. In addition, there have been more than a few cases of contaminants appearing in supplements, particularly in amino acids and mood-enhancers such as tryptophan. These can cause a host of problems. You vastly improve your chances of getting a quality product by selecting a major manufacturer's brand.

Don't megadose. Taking too much of a vitamin or supplement can be dangerous. For example, fat-soluble vitamins, such as A and D, can be toxic in large amounts (do not exceed doses of 10,000 IU of Vitamin A or 50 mcg of vitamin D), causing liver and kidney damage and other problems. Taking too much of a trace mineral, such as zinc, copper, selenium, or magnesium, can impair your absorption of other nutrients.

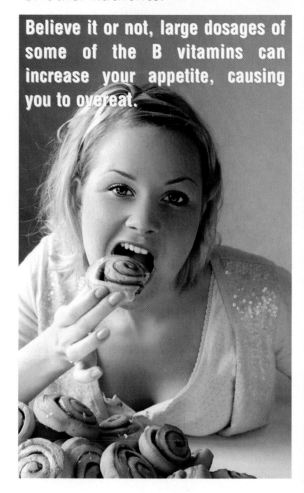

Believe it or not, large dosages of some of the B vitamins can increase your appetite, causing you to overeat.

Athletic Supplements

You may not consider yourself an athlete. You may not think that you will *ever* be an athlete. However, **once you begin walking regularly you may decide you want to start jogging.** Once you start jogging you may decide you want to enter a local 5k. Once you've run a 5k you may say to yourself, "Perhaps next year I can place better." Believe me, this can happen to the most non-athletic person! So here is a small sample of supplements proven to help with athletic endeavours.

Glutamine

Glutamine is the most abundant amino acid in the human body and is considered conditionally essential. This means that, **while the body can manufacture it, there** are times when demand outstrips synthesis rates (stress and exercise being just two of the occasions).

Glutamine plays a very important role in protein metabolism, and it appears to be very important for serious athletes. In hard-training athletes, muscle deterioration can occur because **tissues that need glutamine will rob the muscles of their store.** Not only athletes, but also those who have been under a lot of stress or trauma (such as burn, surgery, and disease victims) can really benefit from glutamine supplementation.

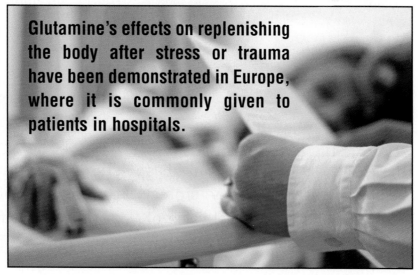

Glutamine's effects on replenishing the body after stress or trauma have been demonstrated in Europe, where it is commonly given to patients in hospitals.

Whey Protein

When cream is separated to make cheese, the remaining liquid is called whey. Whey is almost completely made up of protein. Long considered a useless by-product of cheese manufacturing, whey at one time was considered a "disposal problem" by the dairy industry. But no longer. Research over

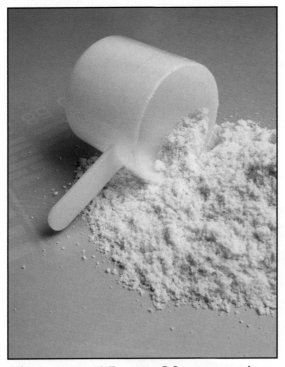

the past 15 to 20 years has demonstrated that whey protein has the highest biological value of any protein. The dairy industry now makes a profit selling something that used to be thrown away.

Whey has become such a popular athletic supplement because it's rich in certain amino acids and low in fat. Some of the amino acids, called the branched-chain amino acids (leucine, valine and isoleucine) may help delay fatigue during endurance exercise. Whey is also high in glutamine. Finally, whey is very easy to mix and doesn't seem to cause the digestive problems of many of the other protein supplements. A couple of swirls with a spoon and your protein drink is ready. No need for blending.

Creatine

Creatine is the most popular supplement currently available. Since its first release in the mid 1990s it has taken the athletic world by storm. **Creatine is also one of the few supplements to have good scientific evidence to back up its effectiveness.**

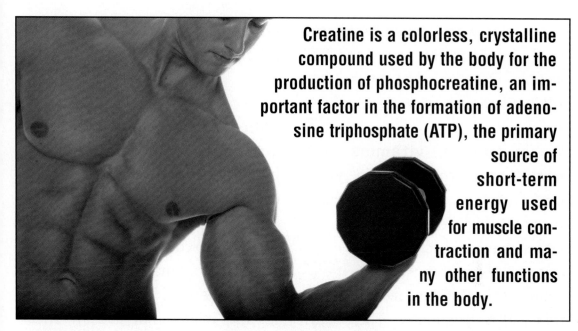

Creatine is a colorless, crystalline compound used by the body for the production of phosphocreatine, an important factor in the formation of adenosine triphosphate (ATP), the primary source of short-term energy used for muscle contraction and many other functions in the body.

Vitamins and Minerals

Vitamins are essential substances that your body uses to do hundreds of things, from growth and development to preventing the cellular oxidation that causes cancer. You need vitamins to help with blood clotting and energy production. Vitamins are even involved in making sure you can see in color. They play a major role in keeping your immune system healthy. It's safe to say that at least one vitamin is involved in every metabolic reaction in the human body.

Fat- and water-soluble

There are two types of vitamins: fat-soluble and water-soluble. When you eat foods that contain fat-soluble vitamins, the vitamins are stored in the fat tissues in your body and in your liver for later use. Fat-soluble vitamins may remain stored in your body for days or even months. Then, when they are needed, special carriers take them. **Because they can be stored, it is possible to build fat-soluble vitamins up to toxic levels by supplementing.** While the amounts in a one-a-day vitamin tablet won't cause problems, don't megadose on any of the fat-soluble vitamins. The major fat-soluble vitamins are A, D, E, and K.

Water-soluble vitamins are not stored for long in your body. Instead, they travel quickly through your bloodstream and are either used or excreted when you urinate. For this reason these types of vitamins need to be replinished frequently. The major vitamins in this group include vitamins C and the big group of B vitamins: B1 (thiamin), B2 (riboflavin), niacin, B6 (pyridoxine), folic acid, B12 (cobalamine), biotin, and pantothenic acid.

Minerals

Like vitamins, minerals are extremely important for such metabolic processes as growth, repair, and fighting of infections. **The body uses minerals to perform many different functions, from building strong bones to transmitting nerve impulses, from muscle contraction to regulating the heart beat.**

Macro and Trace

There are two kinds of minerals: macrominerals, usually just called minerals, and trace minerals, usually called trace elements. Macro means "large" in Greek (and your body needs larger amounts of macrominerals than trace minerals). The macromineral group is made up of calcium, phosphorous, magnesium, sodium, potassium, chloride, and sulfur.

Just because the word "trace" appears doesn't mean trace elements are less important than macrominerals. Your body needs them just as badly, just not in the same quantities. The trace mineral group includes iron, manganese, copper, iodine, zinc, cobalt, fluoride, and selenium.

You really cannot overestimate the importance of vitamins and minerals. A proper diet that includes plenty of produce, and a daily multivitamin/mineral tablet will go miles toward keeping you looking and feeling great.

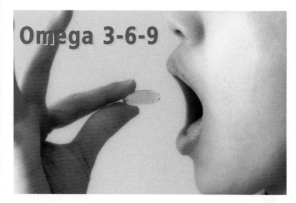

Omega 3-6-9

Every day seems to bring more information about the benefits of "The Omegas," omega 3 fatty acid in particular. While eating foods rich in omega 3 (oily fish such as salmon; nuts, flaxseed) is essential for good health, supplementing with fish oil is never a bad idea.

Omega 3 has been shown to help with all these conditions:
- **Depression**
- **Cardiovascular disease**
- **Type 2 diabetes**
- **Fatigue**
- **Dry, itchy skin**
- **Brittle hair and nails**
- **Inability to concentrate**
- **Joint pain**

In addition (and ironically) taking **fish oil and other rich oily sources of omega 3 helps to keep you lean!**

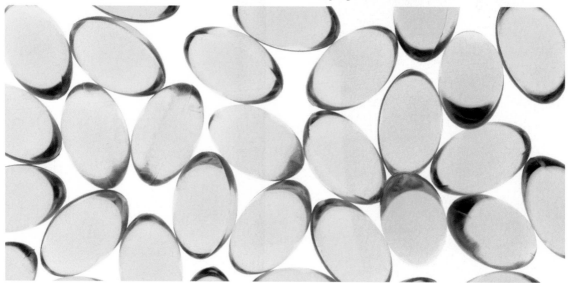

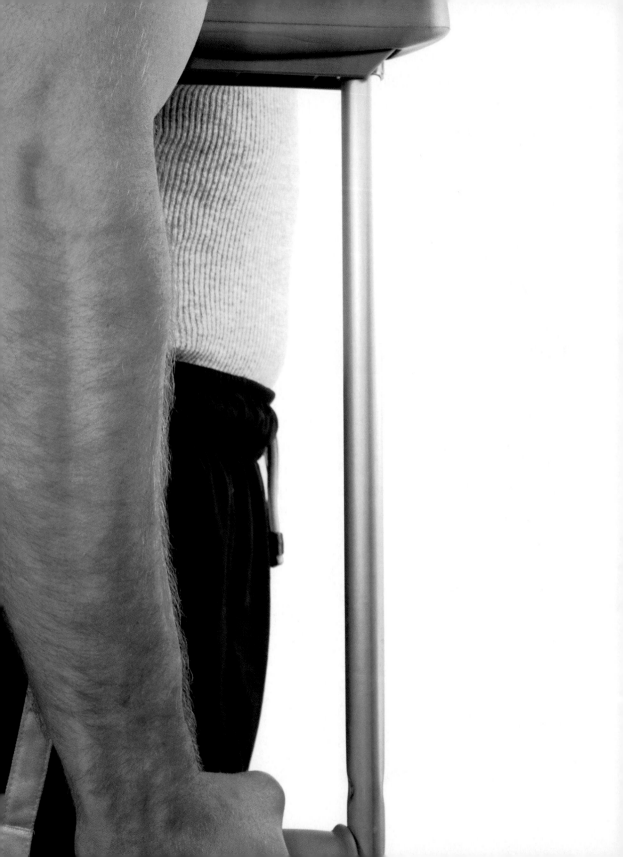

Chapter 10
INJURIES

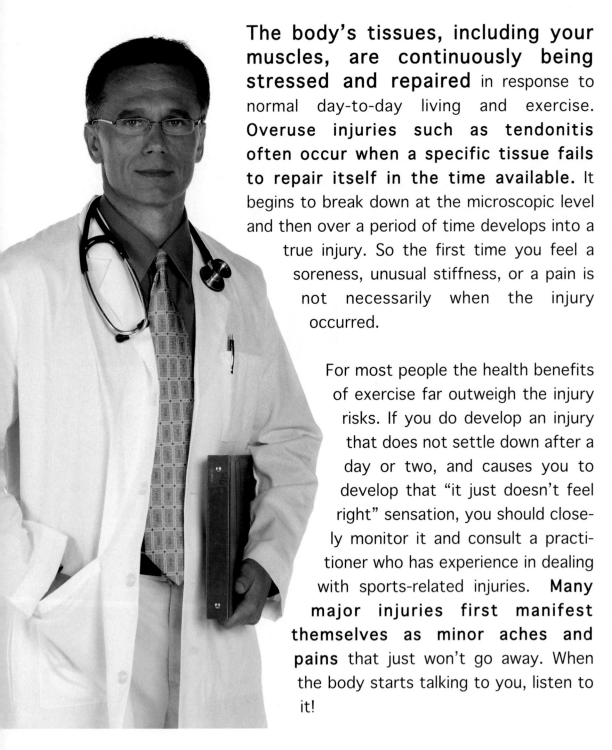

The body's tissues, including your muscles, are continuously being stressed and repaired in response to normal day-to-day living and exercise. Overuse injuries such as tendonitis often occur when a specific tissue fails to repair itself in the time available. It begins to break down at the microscopic level and then over a period of time develops into a true injury. So the first time you feel a soreness, unusual stiffness, or a pain is not necessarily when the injury occurred.

For most people the health benefits of exercise far outweigh the injury risks. If you do develop an injury that does not settle down after a day or two, and causes you to develop that "it just doesn't feel right" sensation, you should closely monitor it and consult a practitioner who has experience in dealing with sports-related injuries. Many major injuries first manifest themselves as minor aches and pains that just won't go away. When the body starts talking to you, listen to it!

Causes of Injury

Following are some of the common causes for injuries. This section is not to be used as a self-diagnostic manual. **At the first sign of an injury, play it safe and consult your physician.**

Constant repetition

This is probably the most common cause of minor injuries. The primary difference between walking and running is that in walking there is always one foot on the ground whereas in running there is a point where neither foot is in contact with the ground. This means that running is a series of leaps or jumps from one leg to the other and so the stresses are so much greater. And, unlike weight training, where the extra stress is on the muscles and soft tissues only for about 30 seconds or so, you could be running for 30 minutes or more.

Poor style

The way you exercise can play a big role in injury prevention. This is especially the case with running. Running slouched, arched, or knock-kneed can all affect your efficiency and therefore the poten-

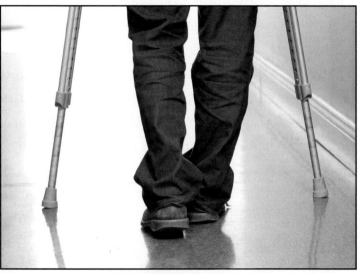

tial for developing a serious injury.

If you feel your style may be irregular, you could be setting yourself up for an injury down the road. Consult a coach or trainer who has experience with working with athletes before you go about trying to change things on your own.

Inadequate recovery

All forms of exercise place stress on the body. If given adequate rest and time to recover, this stress will stimulate the body to adapt in a positive manner, making it stronger and healthier. However, if adequate sleep or time between training sessions is not allowed, the body is not able to recover fully. This can result in minor damage to soft tissues, and if they are not fully repaired they may be damaged further during subsequent training sessions. Over time numerous little problems can add up to one big problem. This is how most overuse injuries occur.

Always allow adequate time for adequate recovery before starting to exercise again.

Poor nutrition

Muscle glycogen is an essential fuel during strenuous exercise, and during intense training sessions it is rapidly depleted. Once it depletes, exercise performance is impeded. **Glycogen stores are replenished by eating plenty of carbohydrates.** If you don't adequately replenish your glycogen stores, you'll be starting your next workout in a semi-depleted state. This will lead to early fatigue, poor style, and therefore an increased

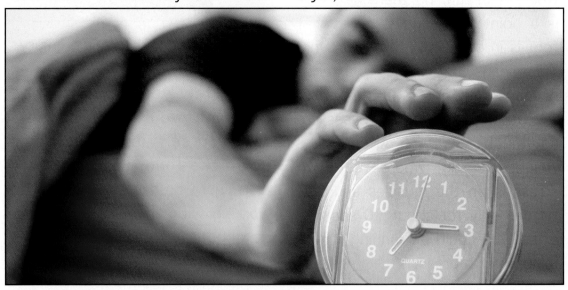

risk of injury. **Nutrition should be treated with as much respect as training and footwear.**

Inappropriate training

As everyone is unique it's not surprising that we'll all respond differently to training programs. Even people with similar builds and fitness levels may need different programs to get the most out of their workouts. What works for one may not work for someone else. For example, running in a group can be very beneficial for motivation, but if you spend your whole run trying to catch up to everyone else, you will soon find yourself in a state of overtraining. Your program must involve appropriate intensity levels, duration, and frequency, so adaptation occurs gradually and with subsequent strength and fitness gains.

Not ready

Also be extra careful when resuming training following injury or illness. We often convince ourselves that we are ready for a certain session when really we are not. The risk of injury is always looming around the corner if we push things too hard too fast.

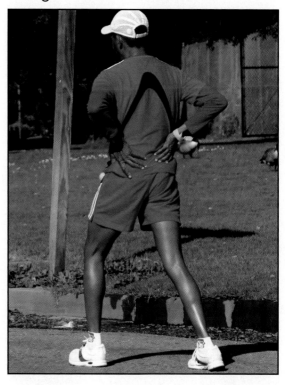

Always try to have a clear idea as to the goal of that training session. **There is no disgrace in starting at a lower intensity level** or with a shorter session to ensure that the workout doesn't inhibit your recovery.

Adapt

You have your training program all planned out. **Consistency is the key to success, but sometimes you have to give in to your body's needs.** Be honest with yourself. If you're feeling "under the weather," you might want to do an easy workout, or possibly skip it altogether. The most successful (and injury-free) athletes are those who are not afraid to adapt their plans according to how they feel where appropriate.

Pre-existing postural and anatomical concerns

Certain postures and anatomical factors can predispose a runner to injury. For example, if one leg is slightly longer than the other (more common than you think) this could stress the lower back, hips, knees, and shins. Go to a sports medicine clinic and most of these concerns can be easily addressed.

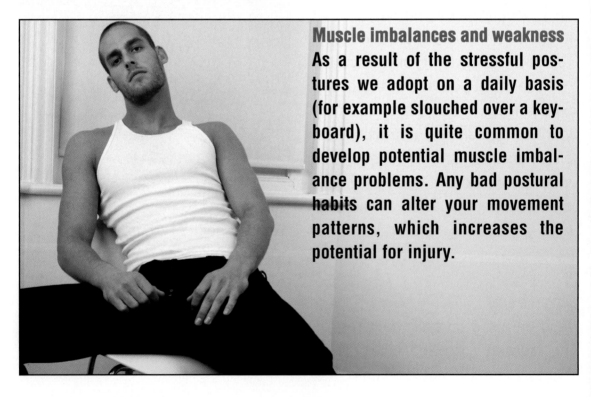

Muscle imbalances and weakness

As a result of the stressful postures we adopt on a daily basis (for example slouched over a keyboard), it is quite common to develop potential muscle imbalance problems. Any bad postural habits can alter your movement patterns, which increases the potential for injury.

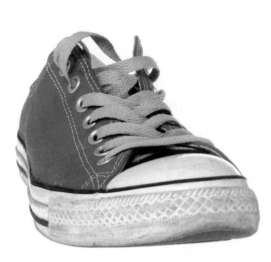

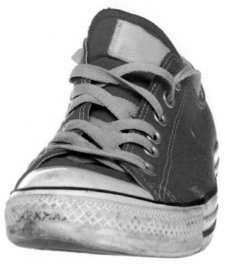

Prior injury

Runners are notorious for thinking that they have fully recovered from an injury when the pain is reduced enough to allow them to resume running. But even when most of the pain is gone, such other injury-related issues as tightness, weakness, and imbalances may still persist. Failure to accept that rehabilitation often has to continue on after the pain is gone can leave a runner ripe and ready for redeveloping the injury, or worse: sustaining a more serious injury.

Inappropriate footwear

Even though we covered this early in the book, it needs repeating here. Proper shoes, appropriate to the chosen sport and to the size and weight of the person, are a vital component in injury prevention. Your running shoes should be regularly checked for signs of excessive wear. Check for wear on the outer sole, breakdown of the mid-sole, distortion of the heel region, and damage to the upper sections of the shoe.

Types of Injuries

Just about every tendon, ligament, or muscle on the human body is a site for a potential injury. As this book is primarily aimed at runners, we'll discuss the injuries that this group of exercisers occasionally fall victim to.

Shin splints

Shin splints is a catch-all term for a number of conditions that can cause lower leg pain. As with all muscles, the muscles of the lower leg are surrounded by a thin restraining membrane called fascia. Both the muscles and fascia are attached to the tibia and fibula (lower leg bones). **Repetitive movements such as running sometimes cause the fascia to become inflamed.**

Symptoms
Generally speaking, minor pain will initially occur in the lower legs the morning after an intensive running session. In most cases the pain will subside, but if it persists and intensifies it will limit the level of future activity.

Causes
Shin splints have numerous causes, including increased levels of running, poor footwear, prolonged running on hard surfaces, poor running style, or tight lower leg muscles.

The muscles will initially work harder to try to help control your running motion. This often leads to soreness because of inflammation to the surrounding fascia or tendons. With continued activity, the muscles will place additional stress on the fascia, which will pull at its attachment on the bone. This can cause the outer edge of the bone to become extremely sore and tender. With continued activity the soft outer layer of the bone will become inflamed. In severe cases, a stress fracture may occur, which is a small break in the bone often not visible on X-ray.

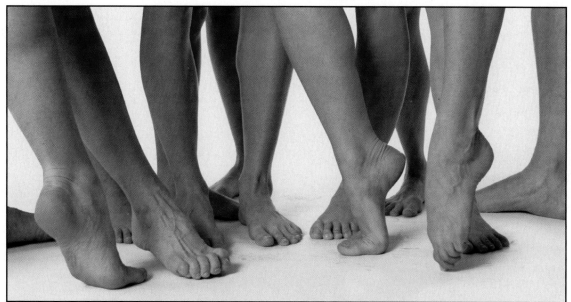

What you can do

All of these symptoms can be reduced or eliminated by a combination of rest, reducing the activity, running on softer ground, and improving your footwear. If there is no improvement or things get worse, seek medical advice.

What they can do

Physiotherapy, including stretching and strengthening exercises, and possibly the fitting of customized shoe inserts may be required.

Average recovery time

The simple answer is one to two weeks. But if you let things go on without addressing the problem, you may require a month or more to fully recover.

Prevention

Obviously it makes more sense to prevent injuries than treat them. The key to preventing shin splints is a combination of doing a proper warm-up, wearing well-fitting footwear, and following a training program appropriate to your fitness level. If you run outdoors, try to avoid hard surfaces, running the exact same route all the time, and suddenly increasing your mileage.

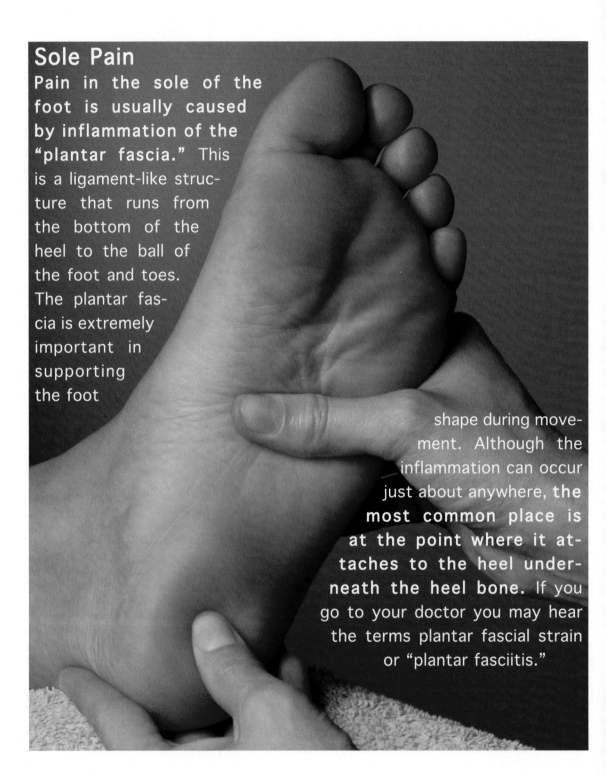

Sole Pain

Pain in the sole of the foot is usually caused by inflammation of the "plantar fascia." This is a ligament-like structure that runs from the bottom of the heel to the ball of the foot and toes. The plantar fascia is extremely important in supporting the foot shape during movement. Although the inflammation can occur just about anywhere, **the most common place is at the point where it attaches to the heel underneath the heel bone.** If you go to your doctor you may hear the terms plantar fascial strain or "plantar fasciitis."

Symptoms

As the name suggests, the symptoms of sole pain are just that: discomfort in the sole of the foot when you place your foot on the ground, especially first thing in the morning.

Initially, the symptoms will ease once you get your circulation up and running, but they'll return with increased levels of activity. **As the condition worsens, pain may be present all the time and prove debilitating.**

Causes

High levels of exercise activity and/or poor foot movement are the most common causes of sole pain, but there is a whole range of other conditions and illnesses that can contribute to similar symptoms.

What you can do

As soon as you notice slight pain in the sole, start stretching the calf muscle. Next increase your rest intervals and apply both heat and ice.

You can give your feet a quick little ice massage by freezing a can of soda pop, covering it with a towel, and rolling your foot over it for 5 to 10 minutes.

Another effective temperature treatment is to alternate submerging your foot in a bowl of warm water for one minute with cold water for 30 seconds. Cushioning the heels with inserts may be beneficial but the inserts may need to be customized by a professional. If your symptoms persist or worsen you should seek a professional opinion.

What they can do

Medical professionals can advise appropriate exercises, strap (to support the foot position), prescribe orthotics, and they sometimes recommend splints that keep the fascia stretched

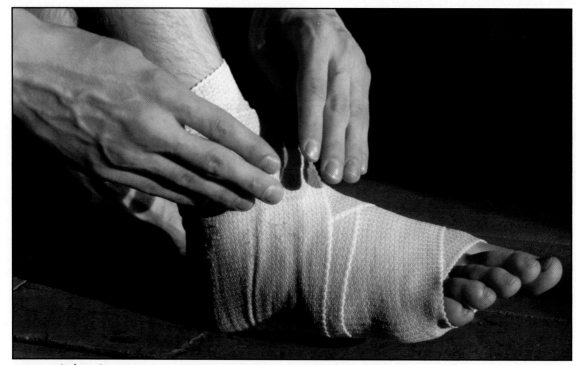

overnight. In more severe cases an anti-inflammatory injection (cortisone) could be needed. As a last resort a cast or surgery may even be required.

Average recovery time
Can be weeks, months, or years.

Prevention
Proper warm-up, good stretching, appropriate footwear, and a training program suited to your fitness levels.

Heel Pain
Heel pain is usually caused by damage to the tissues near the Achilles' tendon, which runs from the bottom of the calf muscles to the upper part of the heel bone. Several conditions can affect the Achilles' tendon causing pain and discomfort.

Symptoms and causes
As heel pain is a complex issue, we're going to separate the causes down into categories.

1. Increased pulling on the tendon where it joins the heel bone (calcaneus) can cause significant discomfort. This condition is called "insertional tendonitis."

2. Bursitis. This is inflammation of the small fluid filled sac (bursa), situated between the Achilles' tendon and the calcaneus.
Note: The symptoms of insertional tendonitis and bursitis are most pronounced in the heel bone region and are particularly painful as the heel lifts from the ground.

3. There can be a buildup of bone material at the back of the heel bone where the tendon attaches. This can cause irritation of the tendon in that area.

4. Paratendonitis. A small sheath called a "paratendon" surrounds the tendon. While the sheath has a good blood supply, the tendon itself has a relatively poor blood supply. This sheath functions to allow the tendon to move smoothly through the tissue, but sometimes the sheath can become inflamed and cause discomfort. In some cases there tends to be a general thickening along the course of the tendon.

5. In cases in which the tendon becomes injured a thickening will occur where the pain is most pronounced. This will cause the area of discomfort to move with the tendon. Surprisingly there will often be less pain when the tendon is under tension than when it's relaxed.

What you can do

The best cure for this is rest from running. When you feel like you've recovered, wait an extra few days and then re-introduce running on alternate days and at a reduced intensity. If possible try to avoid unnecessary walking and stair climbing. You may also want to replace some of your running sessions with other forms of low-impact training.

What they can do

In most cases, medical treatment consists of calf stretches to remove some of the tension, wearing of appropriate shoes, customized orthotics to control the foot position, and physiotherapy. Strengthening some of the other muscles around the ankle can often help relieve symptoms. If there is bony enlargement it may require protective padding. In pronounced cases, surgery may be necessary.

Average recovery time

Two weeks to long term

Prevention

Regular stretching, proper footwear, and appropriate training programs.

Other healing measures:
- Avoid wearing low-support or high-stress shoes such as high-heels.
- Heat the area before running and cool it immediately afterwards.
- Massage the area to increase blood flow and make the region more pliable.
- Stretch the calf muscles well, two or three times each day.
- Use anti-inflammatory skin creams or gels in the area of pain.
- Try putting small heel inserts into your training shoes to reduce the tension on the calf muscles.

Knee Pain

Most knee pain is caused by the inflammation of the knee tendon in the region just below the knee cap (patella). This is called patella tendonitis.

Symptoms

There will be pain and sometimes swelling in the area just below the kneecap. The pain will be most pronounced when tightening the muscles of the front of the thigh, especially as the foot hits the ground.

There may also be pain when you sit for long periods of time with the knee in a bent position.

Causes

The most common causes of knee pain are:

• Poor running technique
• Spinal problems causing muscle movement to be restricted
• Tight muscles
• Weakness, or poor development of certain muscles.
• Extra bone development (called a "spur") in the lower region of the kneecap.

What you can do

• Rest from any activity which irritates the knee for at least two days
• Ice the area of pain for up to 20 minutes every two to three hours
• Regularly massage the area with an anti-inflammatory cream or gel
• Regularly stretch the thigh muscles, hip muscles, glutes, hamstrings, and calves. The stretches should be repeated three times per muscle group and held for at least 15 seconds.

If the pain has not significantly improved after five to seven days, then a consultation with a therapist or doctor who has experience treating running injuries should be sought.

What they can do

Medical professionals can use local electrotherapy and manual therapy techniques such as massage and deep-tissue pressure to improve the quality of the tissue in the region. This will release abnormal tightness from the pelvis down to the knee. It will also correct abnormal biomechanics (i.e. the way in which the leg moves).

Average recovery time

One to three weeks, depending on severity (longer if you allow it to become chronic).

Prevention

• Warm up and stretch appropriately.
• Make use of self- and professional massage.
• Have a biomechanical assessment.
• Avoid poor training practices.

Preventing Injuries

As a runner trying to maximize your health and fitness potential, the risk of injury is very real at any time. But by following the advice laid out in the previous sections of this book, you can reduce if not eliminate the risk of sustaining a serious injury.

At right is a summary of how to prevent and treat minor injuries. But as we keep stressing, at the first sign of something more serious, or if there is any doubt in your mind, contact a medical professional.

General Guidance

As a golden rule, if you feel any degree of tightness, irritation, or pain during or after the training session and it doesn't subside after 24 hours, then resting the next day is the appropriate course of action. If you can still feel it two or three days later, then a trip to a physiotherapist or medical doctor who has experience in dealing with running injuries should be sought.

These suggestions should help you avoid injury:

- Estimate your level of fitness

- Recognize your strengths and weaknesses

- Clearly identify your goals

- Plan an appropriate training program based on the previous three points

- Modify your lifestyle where possible to minimize the negative effects of poor posture, lack of sleep, improper eating, etc.

- Don't be afraid to modify your training approach over time.

- Always train and run in appropriate footwear

- Replace footwear regularly

- Always warm up and cool down

- Always follow a stretching routine

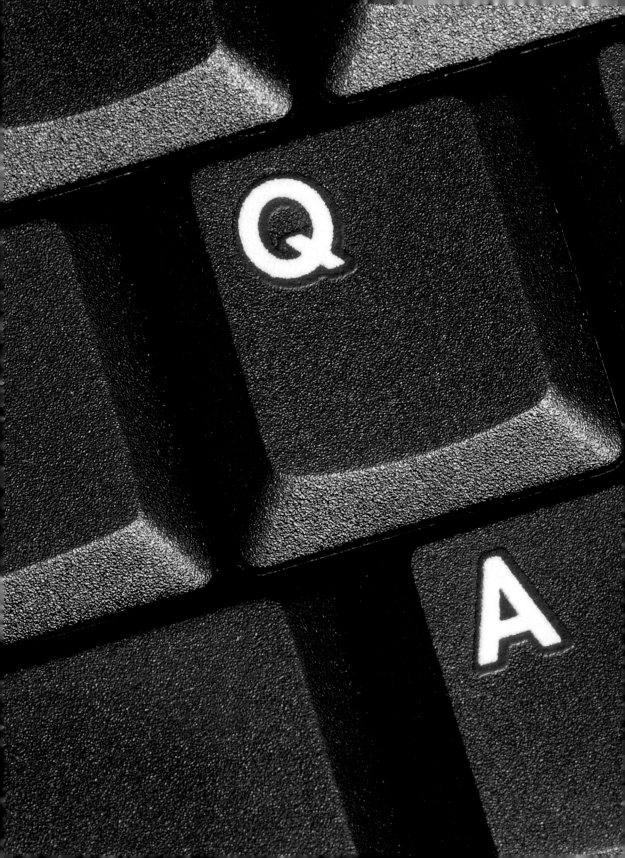

Chapter 11

QUESTION AND ANSWER

My husband maintains that walking on a treadmill is easier than walking the equivalent distance on the ground. He claims this is because the treadmill moves you along the belt somewhat and ground-walking does not. Is this true? **Does walking outdoors burn more calories than walking on a treadmill?**

There is no significant difference in calorie-burning when walking outdoors vs walking on a motorized treadmill. Both forms of exercise will burn approximately the same number of calories per unit time. However, when you run or walk outdoors you have differences in surface levels that force you to use more stabilizing muscles. If you have been running five miles at home with little difficulty you may find five miles outside stresses your system more. If you are planning on entering a race or any kind of a run, it's a good idea to do some of your training outdoors.

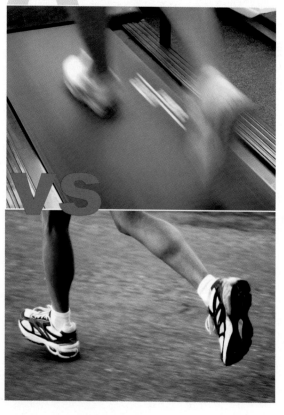

I am a 44-year-old woman who weighs over 200 pounds. **I would like to start exercising, but I'm not sure how long I should exercise and how often.** Do you have any ideas or a workout schedule for beginners who are not exactly in great shape?

Many people would like to start getting more exercise but feel embarrassed or simply don't know where to begin. Your first focus should be on safety. If you've been physically inactive for quite some time, you need to be careful not to overdo it from the beginning.

Always consult with your physician before starting a new exercise program. He or she will likely be thrilled that you're starting to look after yourself, but you want to be sure what your condition is like to take any necessary precautions. Especially if you are overweight, you may have heart trouble, high cholesterol or diabetes and be unaware.

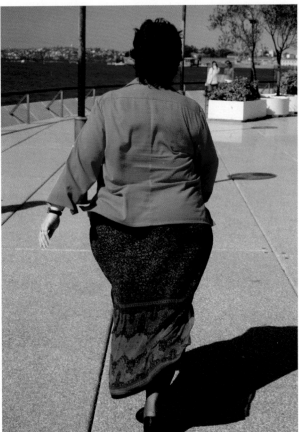

Many people get very excited at the prospect of starting an exercise program, but they wind up doing too much too soon, and quickly burn out. By starting out slowly and being consistent you'll get the results you want and be safe at the same time.

As a suggestion, start off by working out three days per week, going at a comfortable pace that would allow you to carry on a conversation. This is called the "talk test." If you find yourself huffing and puffing and unable to carry on a conversation without long-winded pauses, then you should slow down.

Start out with 15 to 20 minutes walking or keeping an easy pace on the elliptical. If this is too much, try splitting it up.

You might do five minutes, four or five times a day. As you develop your fitness foundation, you can increase the durations and decrease the number of intrrevals.

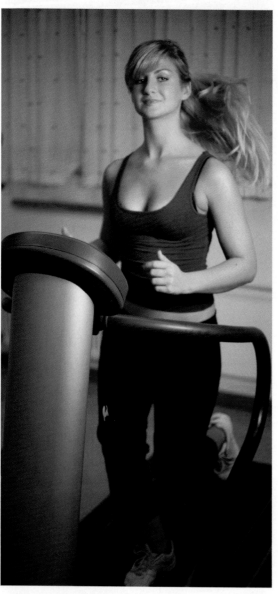

Q Is an elliptical as good as a treadmill for burning fat?

A **Any cardiovascular activity that you can keep up for a substantial period of time will burn fat,** whether that activity is biking, walking, or elliptical training. The main thing, whichever activity you choose, is make sure that you are bringing your heart rate up to the appropriate level for your age and fitness ability.

Q Which is better, running or walking on a treadmill? Also, is it good to use the incline?

A **Neither running nor walking on a treadmill is superior to the other.** As long as the intensity is properly set for your current fitness level (that target heart rate zone again), they will both help you lose weight, and they will both improve your cardiovascular fitness. Walking at a lower intensity for a longer period of time will yield much the same results as running at a higher intensity for shorter periods of time. So you may want to ask yourself how much time you have available in answer to that question. And for this to be true, your walking pace really must be fast enough to get your heart rate up. **Many people stroll rather than walk and then wonder why their weight stays put.**

As for your second question, you'll lose more weight and get into better shape by walking uphill than by walking on a flat surface. Incline walking is as good as running and it's easier on the joints.

Does muscle weigh more than fat? If I am weight training and increasing my muscle mass will I weigh more even though I'm getting in better shape? Should I even weigh myself at all?

This question has been at the center of many debates. The scales tell you only your entire body weight, not your body composi-

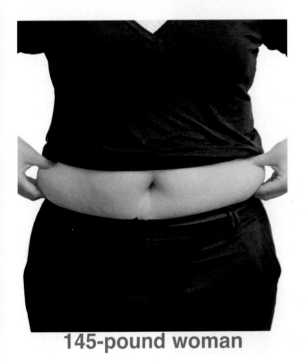

145-pound woman

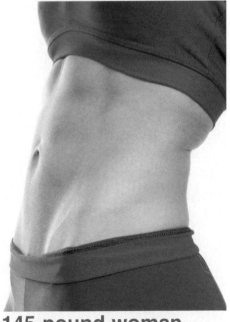

145-pound woman

tion (i.e. the ratio of fat to lean muscle tissue). And **it's body composition that really matters from a health (and beauty) point of view.**

Muscle does not weigh more than fat, any more than lead weighs more than feathers. A pound of feathers weighs the same as a pound of lead. But obviously you'd need a larger volume of feathers to equal a pound than you would lead. The same holds true for fat and muscle. Muscle is much more dense than fat. So **a pound of fat takes up much more space than does a pound of muscle.** In addition, because muscle is biologically active, whereas fat just sits there, increasing your lean muscle mass will help you burn more calories.

Q I have been told that if you consume carbohydrates after 5:00 pm, they'll get stored as fat. Is this true? I'm not losing weight as quickly as I want to.

A The body does not have a fat-burning switch that shuts off at 5:00 p.m. Carbohydrates, especially unrefined complex carbs, don't make you fat; extra calories make you fat, regardless of the time of day you eat them.

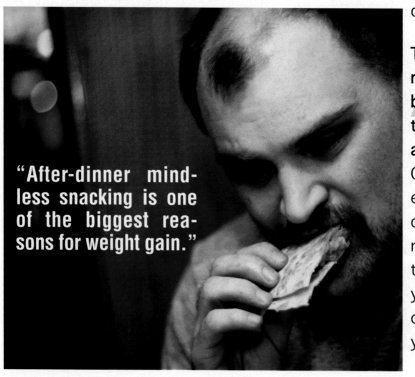

"After-dinner mindless snacking is one of the biggest reasons for weight gain."

Try not to get swept up into the whole high-protein, low-carb fad. These diets may cause short-term weight loss, but they can be dangerous and they certainly cause a lack of energy. In fact, your brain uses glucose (a carbohydrate) as its energy source, so **you may find after depleting carbs for too long that your brain stops functioning properly.**

Now, **this doesn't mean to say you should pig out after 5:00 pm.** After-dinner mindless snacking is one of the biggest reasons for weight gain. Some people consume more calories after dinner than they did the rest of the day. Be conscious of what you put into your body, keep good portion sizes and you really won't have to worry about the time you are eating.

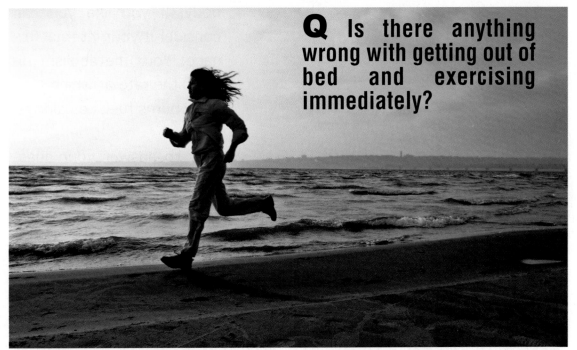

Q Is there anything wrong with getting out of bed and exercising immediately?

There is nothing wrong with exercising just after you wake up. Everyone's biological time clock is a bit different and what works for someone else you may not work for you. If early morning is the time that feels best to you and fits into your daily schedule, then go for it!

As a word of caution, remember that your muscles might be a bit stiff just fresh out of bed, so **make sure that you always do a proper warm-up.** This will help increase your core temperature (which is lowest first thing in the morning) and increase the blood flow to your joints and muscles, all of which helps reduce your risk of injury.

Here's one more consideration concerning morning exercise. Your blood sugar drops throughout the night, and exercising on an empty stomach can really slow you down. **Make sure you eat a small but easily digestible snack before you start your workout.** This will top up your carbohydrate stores and help keep you from crashing after five or ten minutes.

How can I boost my metabolism?

Before talking about speeding up your metabolism, we need to discuss what metabolism is. Simply put, your metabolism is the sum total of all the biochemical reactions taking place in your body. If you like you can consider it your internal furnace. Your metabolism directs the rate at which your body burns fuel, i.e. calories.

Now to answer your question, **the most effective way to speed up and boost your metabolism is through regular physical activity.** You must increase your muscle mass and decrease your body-fat percentage. The best way to increase your muscle mass is through resistance training. The next step is to include regular cardiovascular exercise, at least three or four times per week. This will both stimulate your cardiovascular system and burn any extra calories you consume. **Finally, you must eat clean**. In other words, you must eat a good, healthy diet that includes protein and complex carbs at every meal, and you must eat those small meals every two to three hours throughout the day. If you give your body a steady supply of nutrients, it will not go into starvation mode, and your metabolism will burn brightly.

Can you recommend some good athletic shoes?

Rather than discussing brands, the main thing is for you to find a shoe that fits your needs – and most important, your feet.

Start by deciding what you will use the shoes for. If you're a jogger, find a good fitting pair of running shoes. If you en-

joy activities with side-to-side motion, like tennis, then you'll need to wear a shoe that offers more side support and ankle protection. If you are using an elliptical trainer, then a "cross-training" shoe should be fine. **Seek out an athletic shoe store with knowledgeable sales staff.** For example, most runners' supply stores have at least one staff member who is a serious runner. They will be better able to assist you with proper fit and answer any questions you may have.

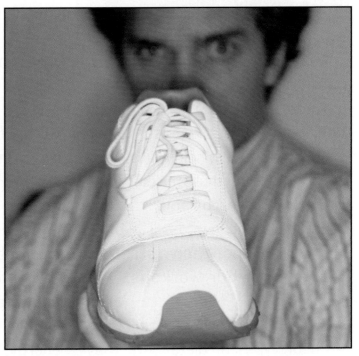

Q Why is it important to warm up before working out?

A In simple terms, warming up prevents injury by making the muscles more flexible. If a muscle is called to work hard when it's cold, the muscle and its attachments are all

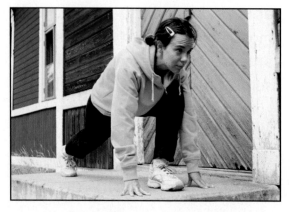

put into a position where they will be more prone to injury. In addition, warming up increases blood supply to muscles, helping to deliver oxygen to the muscles and carry away carbon dioxide and other metabolic wastes. **It's best to warm up, then stretch, then begin your workout.**

Q What's the lowdown on the 24- to 48-hour types of diets? Are they effective for fat loss?

A **These diets are great for two things: dehydrating your body and making you feel sick.** You may lose five pounds, but the five pounds you lose will be water, not fat. Staying on a diet like this for more than two or three days will also cause you to lose valuable muscle tissue. Fat loss, unfortunately, must be done at a slower and more gradual pace. Remember, if it sounds too good to be true it probably is.

Q How long will it take to reach my goal?

A **Goal attainment is dependent on numerous variables** including your exercise experience, age, genetic makeup, time spent training, and the intensity of your training routine. Also understand that the word "goals" can mean different things to each person. For some people feeling better, with more energy, is satisfactory. For others nothing short of a total physique transformation will suffice.

If you have not been engaged in any type of regular exercise, you will definitely feel better after a couple of weeks of physical activity.

Will you lose five inches off your hips in the first week? Probably not. When you see extremely large amounts of weight loss in a very short period of time, the likely reason is dehydration. Only when you are lifting weights, doing cardiovascular exercise three or more times a week, and are on a balanced eating program for at least four to six weeks will you start seeing results.

The best idea is to always have long-term goals and

short-term goals. You may have a short-term goal of walking 0.5 mph more quickly within two weeks, another goal of losing eight pounds within a month, and a long-term goal of fitting into your favorite pair of jeans within six months.

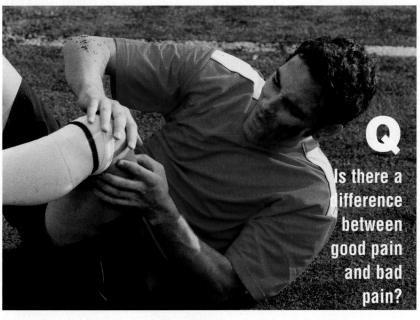

Q Is there a difference between good pain and bad pain?

A Yes! **Good pain should feel symmetrical. That is, both of your arms or legs should have about the same amount of soreness.** Injuries rarely occur in exactly the same place on both sides of the body. Also, the pain shouldn't be deep within a joint. **Good pain should disappear after a couple of days**. Bad pain, on the other hand, is usually non-symmetrical and one side of your body will hurt much more than another. Bad pain will also last much longer - several days or more. If bad pain persists, seek the advice of a doctor.

Q My trainer tells me I should eat after my workout. Why and what should I eat?

A There are two primary reasons why you should eat after exercise; to refuel muscle energy stores, and to supply the nutrients necessary for muscle repair.

During exercise, you burn a mix of fuels including carbohydrate, fats and protein. But the limiting fuel stored in the liver and muscle cells is carbohydrate.

Consuming **carbohydrates and a small amount of protein following exercise assists the body in repairing muscle damage** caused by exercise. To assist recovery (remember, it is during the recovery process that your body improves) you should eat a carbohydrate-rich snack that also contains protein. A protein shake made with milk and containing fruit is an excellent choice.

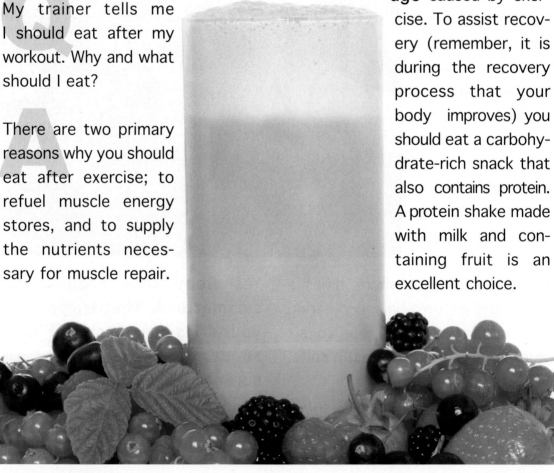

Q Why am I still fat when I eat healthy food and exercise more than my friends? They are lazy and eat junk food but I am still the fat one! Help, I'm only 16 years old!

A People have been fed the story that being overweight is caused only by lack of activity and eating patterns. Yet **genetics also plays a major role in body shape and size.** More than any other age group, teenagers display vast differences in their bodies. Some teens eat thousands of calories of junk food each day while staying lean. Others diet and exercise and always seem a little chubby.

Diet also affects metabolism. **If you have been dieting your metabolism is likely messed up – especially if you are in the habit of skipping meals.** The best way to keep your metabolism burning brightly is to eat small, healthy meals and snacks frequently throughout the day. Teen girls in particular seem to think skipping meals is a good way to lose weight, when **nothing could be further from the truth.**

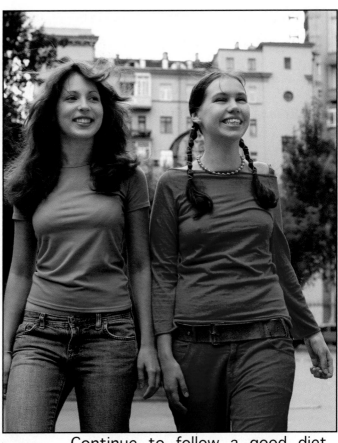

Continue to follow a good diet, eating at least five small meals every two to three hours, keep your active lifestyle, and **you will eventually succeed. Don't give up!**

APPENDIX

RESISTANCE-TRAINING EXERCISES

While this book is not about training with weights (or resistance), weight training causes so many benefits to a person's body that we decided to include a chapter. Resistance training makes you stronger for everyday tasks, it improves balance, helps relieve general aches and pains and raises your metabolism, helping you lose fat and keep it off.

ABDOMINALS

CRUNCHES

Lie face up on the floor with your knees bent and feet flat on the floor. With your hands resting by your sides and your eyes fixed on one point on the ceiling, slowly lift your shoulders about eight to ten inches off the floor. At no time does your butt leave the floor as in a traditional sit-up. Slowly lower back down, stopping one to two inches from the floor.

Now, normally we do not think Swiss balls (inflatable fit balls) are all they've been touted to be. However, for abdominal work they've proven their worth. Tests have shown that contractions of abdominal muscles are stronger when crunching on a fit ball than when crunching on a mat.

COMMENTS – Most people

consider crunches one of the best abdominal exercises. At first you may want to perform the movement with your hands by your sides. As you get stronger, place your hands to the side of the head – doing so adds the weight of the arms to your upper body, making the exercise more difficult.

MUSCLES INVOLVED – Crunches work the rectus abdominis. The exercise also brings the hip flexors into play, athough to a much lesser extent than sit-ups.

REVERSE CRUNCHES

Lie on your back on the floor and extend your legs straight out in front of you. With your upper body held stationary, slowly draw your knees toward your torso, trying to keep your lower legs parallel with the floor. Slowly stretch your legs back out to just short of a lockout.

COMMENTS – To reduce the stress on the lower back, never let your legs completely lock out. Always keep a slight bend.

MUSCLES WORKED – Although the upper abs receive some stimulation, reverse crunches primarily target the lower abs. The hip flexors also come into play.

◀◀◀◀◀◀   **KNEE RAISES**

Hang from a chinning bar. You can either hold on with your hands or use straps made for this purpose. Stretch your legs down and then lift your knees toward your chest. Try not to swing. Use slow controlled movements. As your abdominal strength improves you can try doing this exercise with straight legs. When you can do 3 sets of 25 reps your abdominals will be very strong.

COMMENTS – Resist the urge to use your upper body to pull your legs up. Use only abdominal strength.

MUSCLES WORKED – Knee and leg raises primarily work the lower abdominals, but the upper abs and hip flexors also come into play.

LEGS

SQUATS

Place the barbell on the squat rack, about shoulder height. Step under the bar and rest it across your shoulders. Step back, away from the rack, and place your feet just slightly wider than shoulder width apart. Now in a slow and controlled manner bend your knees and descend towards the floor. Stop when your thighs are approximately parallel with the floor. Pause for a second and then return to the starting, upright position.

COMMENTS – Most consider squats to be the king of the thigh exercises. If done properly they do wonders for toning and strengthening your legs. Done improperly they may put you in traction. Don't bounce at the top or bottom of the exercise. Remember, you have a loaded barbell on your shoulders, which is putting a lot of stress on your spine. Keep control of the weight throughout the movement.

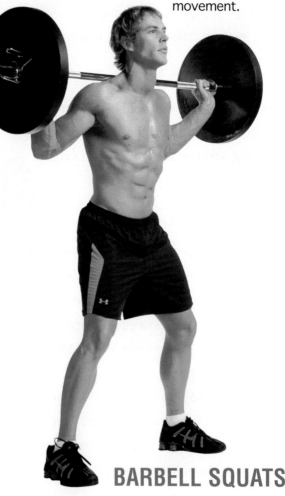

BARBELL SQUATS

Make sure you rest the bar across your shoulders and traps, not on the bony protrusion at the base of your skull. Do so and you will need regular chiropractic visits!

MUSCLES WORKED – While primarily a quad exercise, squats will stimulate the whole leg and glute (buttock) region. Also, the calves and hamstrings are used in stabilizing the legs as you move up and down. The wider the stance, the more glute involvement

Finally, and much less obviously, the spinal erectors (lower back muscles) are needed to keep the body upright. In fact they are often the weak link in the chain.

Most injuries obtained while doing squats center around the lower back region. This is why you must concentrate when performing this exercise. (And strengthen your back!)

LUNGES

Rest a barbell on your shoulders as in the squat, or hold dumbbells in your hands. Slowly step forward and downwards with one leg until there is a 90-degree angle at the knee. Your trailing leg should always have a slight bend at the knee. Return to the standing, upright position.

COMMENTS – You can complete all the reps for one leg and then switch, or

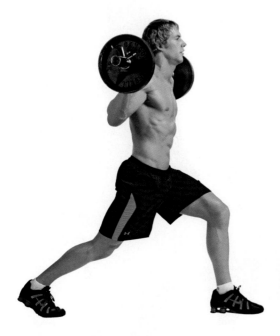

LUNGES

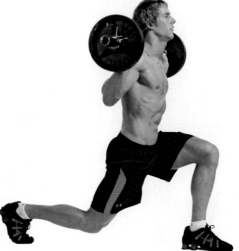

alternate legs on a rep-by-rep basis. Keep your torso erect at all times. Never allow your front knee to move out over your toes, and don't allow the knee of the trailing leg to touch the floor.

MUSCLE WORKED – Lunges work the thighs and glutes, but the hamstrings also come into play.

LEG EXTENSIONS

If you've ever had a sports-related knee injury, this exercise is probably familiar. Leg extensions are among the most popular rehabilitation exercises. Sit down at the machine and place your feet under the padded rollers. Raise the legs to a locked position and squeeze the thighs. Lower back to the starting position and repeat.

COMMENTS – Most home

gyms have a machine that incorporates both the leg (hamstring) curl and leg extension. In other words, you can perform both exercises on the same machine. The same weight stack is used, but for leg extensions you sit on the end and use the lower rollers. For leg curls you lie face down and use the upper rollers. Resist the tendency to drop the weight into the starting position. For variety, you can perform the exercise one leg at a time.

MUSCLES WORKED – Extensions are ideal for building the quadriceps muscles around the knee area. They're also a very effective physiotherapy exercise.

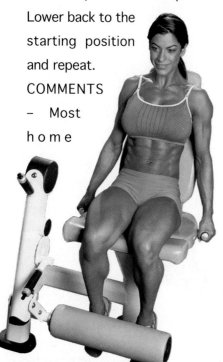

LEG EXTENSIONS

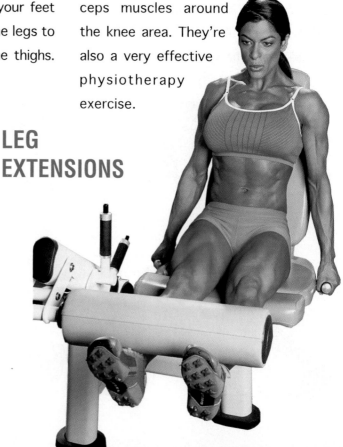

HAMSTRING CURLS

You may find a machine devoted strictly to hamstring curls which has you lying down, as shown, you may find a seated or standing hamstring curl machine or, as we stated earlier, you may find a machine that combines leg extensions and hamstring curls.

COMMENTS – Be careful not to use too much weight, otherwise you risk both straining the lower back and damaging the hamstring muscles. A hamstring tear is quite common. Though this means you should be cautious while performing this exercise, it also means the exercise is especially important – strong hamstrings help prevent that injury from occcuring when you run or do other exercises.

You should concentrate on keeping your toes pointed throughout the exercise rather than keeping your ankle flexed. This helps you target the hamstring muscles as opposed to having the calves help out.

MUSCLE WORKED – The hamstring muscles are the main focus. The calves help out and the glutes are also involved. You can make this more of a glute exercise if you desire: bring the pad up in a curl, then concentrate on pushing your leg back from the hip.

DUMBBELL CALF RAISES

Stand on a block of wood or the bottom step of your stairs. Lift one leg off the floor by bending the knee. Hold a dumbbell in the opposite hand. Slowly stand up on your tiptoes, then stretch down as far as you can comfortably – not till it hurts!

COMMENTS – You will only get good results from calf training if you also get a *good* stretch.

HAMSTRING CURLS

Don't bounce at the bottom. You would risk injuring your Achilles' tendon.

MUSCLES WORKED – Dumbbell calf raises primarily work the gastrocnemius (the muscle we think of as the calf), but the soleus does come into play.

CHEST

FLAT BENCH PRESSES

(Note: Bench presses can all be done with either a barbell or dumbbells.)

Lie on your back and take the barbell from the supports, using a grip that is six to eight inches wider than shoulder width. Lower the bar slowly to the lower chest, and then press it back to the locked-out position.

COMMENTS – King of the chest exercises, bench presses are performed by virtually everyone. A few points to consider: Don't drop the bar and bounce it off the chest. Yes you can lift more weight this way, but you are robbing the exercise of its effectiveness. You also run the risk of breaking ribs or splitting your sternum. Dropping the bar in a loose fashion also increases the risk of tearing the area where your chest muscles connect to your shoulder muscles. Lower the weight in a slow, controlled manner, and then push it back to arms' length.

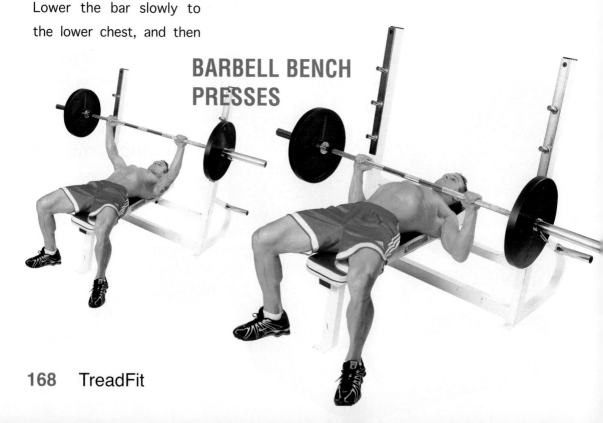

BARBELL BENCH PRESSES

Don't arch your back off the bench. Once again you may increase your lift by a few pounds, but at what cost? Arching decreases the amount of pectoral stimulation, and it certainly is no benefit to your lower back.

If you have trouble keeping your back on

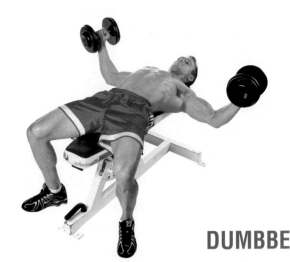

DUMBBELL FLYES

the bench, perform the movement with your legs up in the air or on the bench. You will not be able to use as much weight, but there is no way you can arch your back when in this position.

MUSCLES WORKED – Flat bench presses primarily work the lower chest region, but the whole pectoral-deltoid area is stimulated. You will also find your triceps receiving a great deal of stimulation. Finally, the muscles of the back and fore-

arm are indirectly used for stabilizing the upper body during the exercise.

DUMBBELL FLYES

Start this exercise in the same position as dumbbell presses. Instead of having the dumbbells pointing end to end, rotate your hands until the palms are facing and the dumbbells are parallel with your body. With your elbows slightly bent, lower the dumbbells for a full stretch. Pause at the bottom, and then squeeze the dumbbells up and together, over the center of the chest.

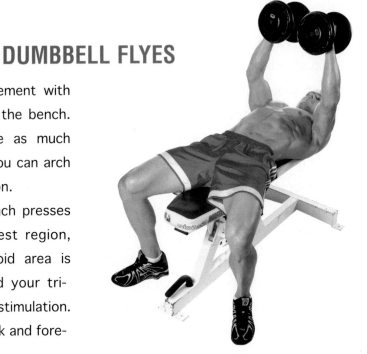

COMMENTS – Flyes are a great stretching and shaping exercise. Always lower the dumbbells in a controlled manner, no matter what weight you are using. Drop them too fast and you'll rip the pec-delt tie-in. Treatment for such an injury is surgery and many months of rehabilitation.

MUSCLES WORKED – Flyes work the whole chest region. Fully stretching at the bottom works the outer chest region and squeezing together at the top develops the inner chest. As there will be some pec-delt tie-in strain, be careful at the bottom of the movement.

INCLINE PRESSES

If using an adjustable bench, set it to an angle of about 30 degrees. Incline bench presses are performed in the same manner as flat bench presses, the only difference being instead of lowering the bar to the nipple region, you should bring it down to the center of the chest just under the chin.

COMMENTS – Most people find angles above 30 degrees place too much stress on the front delts, and not the upper pectorals. Of course your bone structure may dictate the opposite. You may have to play around with the bench's angle to see what works best for you.

MUSCLES WORKED – The incline barbell press primarily works the upper chest. It also stresses the front delts and triceps. Remember, as you increase the angle, the stress shifts from the upper chest to the shoulders.

PEC DECK

Sit down in the machine's chair with your back braced against the vertical back support. Depending on the model, either grab the handles or rest your elbows and forearms against the two arm pads. Slowly squeeze your arms together in a hugging type motion to just short of touching the handles or pads in front. Slowly return the handles or pads back to a comfortable stretch (for most people the arms will be in line with or just slightly behind the shoulders).

COMMENTS – Always keep control of the handles or pads as you are lowering the weight back down. If you bounce at the bottom you run the risk of injuring your shoulder joint.

MUSCLES WORKED – Pec decks primarily work the chest, but the front shoulders also come into play. And unlike most chest exercises that also work the triceps, the pec deck stimulates the biceps to some degree.

BACK EXERCISES

BENT-OVER BARBELL ROWS

Bend over at the waist so your upper body is just short of parallel with the floor. Grab a standard barbell, and using a wide grip, pull it up to the abdomen. Lower slowly and then repeat. Concentrate on using your lats and not your spinal erectors.

COMMENTS – Make sure your back is not rounded! Doing the exercise with a rounded back puts your lower back in a precarious position. To help you to keep an arched back, look up, as shown in the illustration at right. You must be especially careful on this exercise. Any sudden bouncing or jerking will put great stress on your lower back. If you have to "throw your lower back into it," you are using far too much weight. The only part of the body that should move is the arms. Your upper body and legs should remain sta-

tionary.

As a final point, bend your knees slightly. This will help reduce the stress on your lower back.

MUSCLES WORKED – This exercise is considered by most to be one of the best back builders. It's particularly effective in producing thickness in the back. Besides the back muscles, bent-over rows stress the biceps and forearms. Finally, because of the bent-over position, the exercise stretches the hamstrings and spinal erectors.

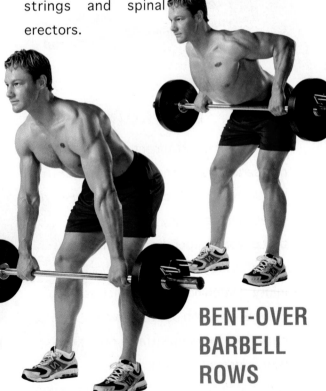

BENT-OVER BARBELL ROWS

ONE-ARM DUMBBELL ROWS

Instead of using a barbell or cable, you can do your rows using a dumbbell. Lean on a bench for support. Grab a dumbbell with your other arm and stretch it down and slightly forward. Pause at the bottom and then pull the dumbbell up until the arm is ful-

ONE-ARM ROWS

ly bent. The movement is comparable to sawing wood.

COMMENTS – One-arm rows are great because they allow you to brace your upper body. This is essential if you have a lower back injury. Even though your biceps will be involved in the exercise, try to concentrate on using just your back muscles. Once again, no bouncing or jerking the weight. If you have to contort the body to lift the weight, the dumbbell is too heavy.

SEATED PULLEY ROWS

You will need a cable machine to perform this exercise. Grab the V-shaped pulley attachment and sit down on the floor or associated board. With the legs slightly bent, pull the hands into the lower chest/upper abdomen. Pause for a second and squeeze the shoulder blades together. Now bend forward and stretch the arms out fully.

COMMENTS – You can perform this exercise with a number of different pulley attachments. The most frequently used is the V-shaped double handle bar. Some people like to use a straight pulldown bar. Others use two separate hand grips. Our advice is to experiment with the different attachments to select the one that feels most comfortable. Cable rows can also be performed on the lat pulldown machine.

To get the full effect, lean back and pull the hands to the lower chest. The direction of force should be about 90 degrees to the body. When doing the seated version, keep the legs slightly bent. Performing the exercise with straight legs will only affect your lower back.

MUSCLES WORKED – Seated pulley rows are another exercise that works the whole back region; although they are more of a center back exercise than outer back movement. As with other rowing exercises, seated pulley rows also stimulate the biceps and forearms.

LAT PULLDOWNS

Sit down on the machine's chair and grab the overhead bar with a slightly wider than shoulder-width grip. Slowly pull the bar down to your chin. Return the bar to the starting position with your arms stopping just short of a lockout.

COMMENTS – Although some people perform the exercise by bringing the bar behind their head, pulling the bar behind the head puts stress on the rotator cuff (the small muscles and tendons located on your shoulder blade). Pulling to the front stimulates the same muscles with much less stress.

MUSCLES WORKED – Front pulldowns work the large latissimus dorsi muscles, the teres, rhomboids, and rear shoulders. They also work the biceps to some degree.

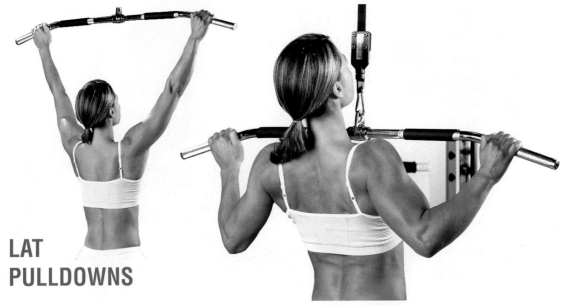

LAT PULLDOWNS

SHOULDER EXERCISES

SHOULDER PRESSES

You'll need something for back support to do this exercise. Most gyms have a proper shoulder press rack, but you can use a chair if you're training at home. Either lift the barbell from the floor and sit in your chair, or reach back and lift the bar off the rack. With a slightly wider than shoulder width grip, slowly lower the bar to your collarbone. Push it back up until your arms are just short of a lock out.

COMMENTS – As with pulldowns, lowering the bar behind the head may over-stress the rotator cuff muscles, so always lower to the front of the head. Also, there is a tendency to arch when doing the exercise, so be careful. A slight arch to bring the bar to the upper chest is fine, but nothing excessive.

MUSCLES WORKED – Front presses put most of the stress on the front and side delts. The triceps also come into play.

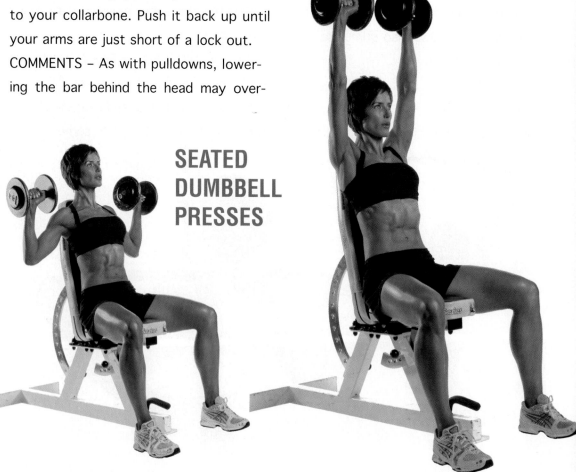

SEATED DUMBBELL PRESSES

DUMBBELL PRESSES

Instead of performing your pressing movements with a barbell, grab two dumbbells and hoist them to shoulder level. You can stand or sit when pressing the dumbbells, but if standing, be careful not to excessively arch the lower back.

COMMENTS – You can press both dumbbells at the same time, or in an alternating fashion. As with the barbell version, be careful of the lower back. Try not to arch excessively, and don't drop the dumbbells into the starting position.

MUSCLES WORKED – This exercise stresses the whole deltoid region. Particular emphasis is placed on the front and side deltoids. There is some secondary rear deltoid and triceps involvement.

UPRIGHT ROWS ▶ ▶ ▶ ▶ ▶

Start the exercise by holding a barbell at arms' length. Using a narrow grip (about three to five inches,) lift the bar up the front of the body, keeping your elbows flared to the sides and the barbell as close to the body as you can get it without it actually touching. Slowly lower to the starting position.

COMMENTS - Which muscles are worked depends on the grip used. Generally speaking, any hand spacing five inches or less puts most of the stress on the side shoulders. Widen the grip and the trapezius comes into play. If you have weak or injured wrists, you might want to think twice about performing this exercise. Upright rows place tremendous stress on the forearms and wrists. If you experience pain when doing the exercise, you may want to skip it.

MUSCLES WORKED - With a narrow grip, upright rows primarily work the side delts. A wide grip shifts the stress to the trapezius. The forearms are worked no matter which grip you use.

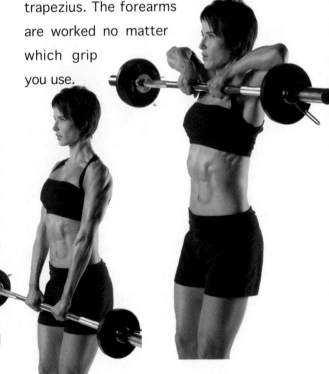

LATERAL RAISES

You can perform this exercise seated or standing. Grab two dumbbells and, with the elbows slightly bent, raise them to the sides of the body. As you raise the dumbbells, gradually rotate the wrists so that the little finger points up. Many authorities, including *MuscleMag International*'s own Robert Kennedy, liken the wrist action to pouring a jug of water.

COMMENTS – You can do the exercise with the arms completely locked, but most people find it more effective to bend the arms slightly and use more weight. Lateral raises can be done to the front, side, or rear. Instead of using dumbbells, a cable may be substituted. Either version may be performed either one or two arms at a time.

MUSCLES WORKED – You can use lateral raises to work any head of the deltoid muscle. Most people do them for the side delts, as the front delts receive ample stimulation from various pressing movements.

FRONT RAISES

The only difference between this exercise and lateral raises is that you lift the dumbbells straight out to the front instead of sideways.

COMMENTS – You may want to experiment with a palms up, palms inward, and palms downward, grip. While all three will target the front shoulder muscles, you may find one more comfortable on the shoulder joint than the others.

MUSCLES WORKED – Front raises primarily target the front shoulders but the side and rear shoulders also come into play.

◄◄◄◄ BENT-OVER LATERALS

This is the bent-over version of regular side laterals. By bending over, the stress is shifted from the side to the rear delts. You can do the exercise standing, seated, or with your head braced on a high bench. The latter is for those with lower-back problems or individuals who have a tendency to swing the weight up.

COMMENTS – Concentrate on lifting the dumbbells with your rear delts and not your traps and lats. For variation try using a set of cables. You will have to grab the cable handles with your opposite hands, so the cables form an X in front of you.

MUSCLES WORKED – When performed properly, bent-over laterals primarily work the rear deltoids. However, the triceps, traps, rhomboids and other muscles are stimulated as secondary muscles.

TRICEPS

ONE-ARM DUMBBELL EXTENSIONS

Grasp a dumbbell and extend it above your head. Keeping your upper arm stationary, lower the dumbbell behind the head. Try to perform the movement in a slow rhythmic manner.

COMMENTS – Keep in mind that the elbow joint and associated tissues (ligaments, cartilage, and tendons) were not designed to support huge poundages, so never bounce the dumbbell at the bottom (arms in the bent position) of the exercise. Try to place the emphasis on style rather than weight.

MUSCLES WORKED – Although it works the whole triceps region, this exercise is especially great for the lower triceps.

LYING DUMBBELL EXTENSIONS

Lie back on a bench and hold a dumbbell in each hand. With the upper arms locked perpendicular the floor, slowly lower the dumbbells to the side of your head. Slowly return to the starting position with your arms locked completely out straight.

COMMENTS – As with any type of dumbbell extension, don't

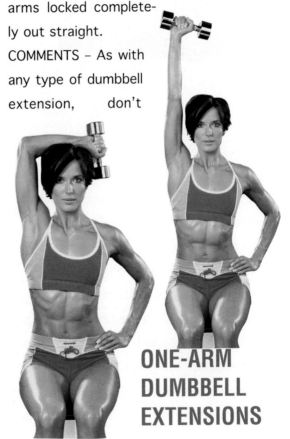

ONE-ARM DUMBBELL EXTENSIONS

bounce the dumbbells at the bottom of the exercise. Try to keep your upper arms locked vertical with the floor.

MUSCLES WORKED – Lying dumbbell extensions work the entire triceps mus-

squeeze at the top, and then lower back to the starting position.

COMMENTS – Resist the urge to swing the dumbbell up using body momentum. True, you can use more weight, but it won't give

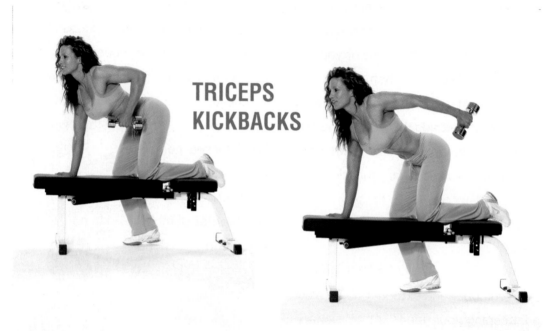

TRICEPS KICKBACKS

cle. The shoulders play a secondary stabilizing role.

TRICEPS KICKBACKS

With your body braced on a bench, bend over and set your upper arm parallel with the floor. Grab a dumbbell and extend the lower arm back until it's in the locked position (i.e. your whole arm is now parallel with the floor). Pause and

the same triceps development. Keep the upper arm locked against the side of the body. As with bent-over laterals, if you have trouble keeping stationary or have a weak lower back, place your free hand on a bench or other such support.

MUSCLES WORKED – Triceps kickbacks are especially useful for developing the long rear head of the triceps.